TANTRIC
YOGA

TANTRIC YOGA

THE ROYAL PATH TO RAISING KUNDALINI POWER

GAVIN AND YVONNE FROST

SAMUEL WEISER, INC.

York Beach, Maine

First published in 1989 by
Samuel Weiser, Inc.
Box 612
York Beach, Maine 03910-0612

99 98
9 8 7 6 5

Library of Congress Cataloging-in-Publication Data

Frost, Gavin.
       Tantric yoga : the royal path to raising kundalini
   power / Gavin and Yvonne Frost.
            p.   cm.
          1. Tantrism—Miscellanea.   2. Yoga—Miscellanea.
      3. Chakras—Miscellanea. 4. Kundalini—Miscellanea.
      I. Frost, Yvonne.   II. Title.
      BF1999.F755   1989
      291.4'48--dc20   89-9128
                                                               CIP
ISBN 0-87728-692-2
CCP

Cover illustration copyright © 1989 Lee Jacobson
Text illustrations on pages 166-244 copyright © 1989 Lee Jacobson

Typeset in 11 point Goudy

Printed in the United States of America

The paper used in this publication meets the minimum requirements of the American National Standard for Permanence of Paper for Printed Library Materials Z39.48-1984.

CONTENTS

ABOUT THE AUTHORS

In the late 1950's Gavin and Yvonne independently researched Eastern religions, avidly reading all available material (see Bibliography). Between 1960 and 1976 Gavin made some fifteen trips to India and Pakistan searching for the remnant teachings of Tantra. Most of the leads he followed turned out to be sexual tourist traps or debased forms of the real teaching that placed great emphasis on the male dominance role and such things as the sacrifice of virgins; but at last in Thailand he found the teaching of John Blofeld. From that start Gavin was able to meet practitioners of a true path in Bengal. After several years of work and experiment, Gavin and Yvonne produced a reconstructed Western Tantra philosophy and life path they believe preserves the essence of the ancient teachings.

In 1985 the School of Wicca offered a course in Tantra. To date over 100 students have completed the course and made their recommendations for changes in the system as taught. The School also invited gays and single practitioners to try the course. Both groups have been successful in achieving spiritual enlightenment.

PREFACE

Many Westerners feel that Eastern religions are so alien as to be of little interest; however, millions who have investigated Yoga have found that even with its exotic language, it can still provide tremendous help toward spiritual development. This book is an advanced text which will introduce you to Reconstructed or Neo-Tantric Yoga, considered by many to be the highest and most rapid path to enlightenment. The book uses very few Sanskrit or Aryan terms. Instead, it uses plain English and symbols, colors, tastes, and all the other sensory keys appropriate to a Western background.

Much of the work in this book is a rediscovery of the old paths. Some of it came through diligent research, some through our own enlightenment, and some from the enlightenment of our students. Typical of these revealed truths are: the interlocking nature of the lunar work/eating/sexual cycles; the inherent quadrality of the Gods and Goddesses and upward and downward creation systems; the underlying meaning of the yin/yang microcosmic in the macrocosm; the reasoning behind the melding of opposites; and a smoother, more natural, and faster path to Nirvana. So far as we can learn, this book reveals these timeless truths in print for the very first time.

We are well aware that the path described in this work will be anathema to Vedic traditionalists, and we expect to hear many fulminations against it. Our intent is not to blaspheme any religion. If we have done so in this work, we wish to apologize now. We have only one justification for revealing this path to the world: *it works*. It may be incomplete. It may just be a light at the end of a tunnel. Yet it is a light after all. If you know a better and easier way, tell us, by at least returning the questionnaire on the last page of the book. Your ideas will help others see more of the light.

A NOTE ON LANGUAGE

We have eliminated foreign words so far as possible, even though to the knowledgeable, the English words we have used in their place are not exact translations. We have retained a few, such as Lingam and Yoni and the names of the God-esses. We have done this because the Western words are either too crude or (in the case of the deities) the Western God-ess names are already culturally loaded. We have also retained some dualistic language and meanings in an attempt to show that certain concepts are not describable in simplistic terminology. Unusual and occasionally strange (supposedly essential) Eastern rituals and exercises have mostly been deleted, since they have been found to be either unnecessary or inhibiting to Westerners. We have retained those that felt natural, though some of these could probably be safely deleted as well. The following list of terms should help you as you continue to study:

Chakra: a center of energy in the etheric body
God-ess: God and Goddess
IT: the Undefinable Ultimate Deity, beyond Shakti and Shiva
Kundalini: the coiled serpent
Lingam mortis: penis in its relaxed state
Lingam vitae: penis erect
Posterior yoni: anus
Prana: the life force
Shakti: the great female archetypal Goddess
Shiva: the great male archetypal God
Yogi: male practitioner of Yoga
Yogin: female practitioner of Yoga
Yoni: vagina

As you go through this book, you will probably be struck by language which seems to be paradoxical. "Clamorous silence," the "singularity of the void," and many similar oxymorons may puzzle you. Some of these paradoxes are quite deliberate. They are meant to awaken your awareness to different concepts. To gain spiritual awareness, you must force your mind into the same type of understanding at a spiritual level. It is possible to comprehend the mind. It is possible to comprehend the spirit that controls the mind. Now your goal is to comprehend the material from which the spirit is made. There is a twofold purpose in paradoxical language:

1) It allows a more exact translation of the original Sanskrit meanings. In many cases the original language has no direct translation into English. The Sanskrit word "citta" is often translated "mind," or sometimes "soul." More correctly, it might be translated as "I"—but the best phrase for it seems to be "the sum of all the attitudes of a conditioned mind" or perhaps "mind reality."

The translation problem has been made significantly worse because of the prudery and bias of the original Victorian translators. Not only did they translate many feminine-gender words (especially goddess names) as masculine; but they also could not comprehend that sexual symbology was meant to serve as a metaphor for spiritual truths. In a time when even table legs had to be covered (literally by a cloth and socially by a euphemism) and a glimpse of ankle was pornographic, those translators went to one extreme or the other. They either gasped in lewd astonishment over the forbidden writing of the Kama Sutra, or suppressed anything vaguely sexual.

2) Paradoxical language allows the mind to grapple with the paradox while the "I" leaves to travel toward the Beyond. The mind knows that it is baffled and must perforce work the problem. The autonomic nervous system keeps the body running; and since the "I" has nothing keeping it in the body, it can leave. This is indeed the path of wisdom; for without the mind that can partially comprehend the paradox and seek for the answer, the system does not work. The mind that totally rejects and

refuses even to try understanding the paradox maintains a firm grip on the body.

It should also be remembered that the only "sins" recognized in the ancient writings are ignorance and ill will.

AN INTRODUCTION TO MODERN TANTRA

Unlike other philosophies, our form of Tantric Yoga encourages its participants to experience the world and its pleasures and thus control their minds so that they can choose to partake or abstain. The esthete abstains from all worldly pleasures and atrophies the senses. The Tantrist believes that after living on bread and water or being celibate for years, the body forgets the exquisite pleasure of the finer things of life and the bodily demand for fulfillment becomes so atrophied that the mind has no difficulty in suppressing the bodily urges. The world of the esthete is full of grays, whereas the Tantrist's world is alive with vivid color.

Nirvana, the ultimate place of serenity and all knowledge, is gained by the Tantrist through a regular cycle of indulgence and abstinence. Through this cyclical training, keyed to the phases of the moon, the Tantrist keeps all the bodily appetites honed to a high degree of sensitivity and the times of abstinence become more and more difficult to endure. Then there is a bursting of the chains, when the mind takes control and Nirvana is achieved.

Tantra is accused by its detractors of being immoral, unethical, and antisocial; but such accusations are completely unfounded. The system is designed to teach a strict (if unusual) moral code, and to develop its adherents spiritually. To achieve such development, the religion requires that both women and men learn to control their passions, and through that ability to gain control of all other body functions, including temperature and pulse rate, and such negative experiences as pain and disease.

Tantra places Woman first; for only through her, it is believed, can Man learn emotional control.

Tantra places great emphasis on discipline, cleanliness, spirituality, and gentleness, but little emphasis on physical beauty. It is negative toward the "love" relationships shown in Hollywood movies. The partner is cherished for proficiency and control in

all ritual matters; other concerns are secondary. If you are looking for perverted practices, you must look elsewhere, for in
Tantra we develop only those activities that are natural and
healthful for both the spirit and the body.

Your daily newspaper blazons across its pages rape, murder,
and mayhem—along with unrealistic descriptions of "beautiful
people." We, on the other hand, glory in the Goddess' gifts to us.
We believe that the human form is one of the highest expres-
sions of Her art. Why clothe it in drab garments or bind it in
unnatural ways in the hope that it will be more provocative to
the opposite gender? Why apply paint and have surgical opera-
tions in the hope that the outward body will be more beautiful,
while ignoring the needs of the inner person and the spiritual
being that dwells tethered to its earthly shell?

Through Tantra we gain complete control of our own emotions, and those around us learn similar control. Some of the
strongest human emotions are those raised by sexual differences.
Once we learn to control them, the lesser emotions—such as
anger and pain—are more easily controlled as well. Students
work through disciplined control toward Nirvana.

When a man sees a beautiful lady or a lady sees a hunk, mild
sexual interest is quite natural; but it is inappropriate to look at
someone and have an actual erection of the nipples, clitoris, or
lingam. The mind is feeding pictures of sexual enjoyment to be
achieved with this desirable person and preparing the body for
the sex act. It would be far better if the mind instead worked out
a clear, logical plan so that, if there is mutual consent, the
desirable person is actually bedded. It is also true that prolonged
sexual arousal will take the edge off the sex act when it finally
happens. Even well-exercised erectile tissue will more quickly
grow flabby after orgasm if it has been erected too early.

You can learn to turn arousal on and off at will, for the
body can be controlled. By some process which we understand
far too little, the fire walker instructs the body that it is not
being damaged by the fire. If the body is under control, indeed it
is not damaged by the fire.

In Tantra, control of the body is ideally learned in a working group. The most fundamental urges, those of procreation and survival, are used to develop the mind's control of the body. High levels of sexual activity with several different experienced partners alternate with proximity but abstinence. Ample food, beautifully prepared, alternates with fasting.

Dedication to the Tantric ideal thus means for instance that lust is indulged, understood, and transcended until all the aspects of genuine love are understood. Climbing the chakras and raising kundalini are used as gauges of this understanding.

Sex is used as one means of traversing the path of control. This use of sex transcends the sexual act, for sex is the *means* by which we obtain transcendence; it is not the end of the road. Copulation and orgasm, beautiful and pleasurable though they are in themselves, do not end with the parting of the copulators but move on, making possible a transition into deep meditation and psychic experience.

Many people use sex to gain their ends. The prostitute and the gigolo get money; the wife might get a new washing machine and the husband a new car. People readily criticize the prostitute and the gigolo, but few criticize the husband and wife; none should criticize the Tantrist. Yet the uninitiated will scorn Tantra as being a path beneath contempt. Jealousy and a feeling of being left out are the main components of such an attitude. Whenever possible it should be ignored; but Tantrists are well warned not to be too public about their affiliation lest they attract negativity.

Someone coming to Tantra as an easy way to get laid will be sadly disappointed, for it may take months to convince a group that you are sincere. Nowadays too, screening for sexually transmitted diseases must be undertaken with great care and patience; many of these lie dormant for months. This often means that a candidate must go through an extended period of celibacy before being admitted to a Tantra house.

To the Tantrist, the ultimate life-style is in a group—what the flower children of the 1960s might have called a group marriage. Couples and individuals can gain immeasurably by practicing the Tantric philosophy; but after reaching spiritual Nirvana, most Tantrists yearn for that all-too-rare experience of living in a Tantra house. This is almost certainly the reawakening of the ancient race memory of close kinship or tribal mutually supportive groups. Through thousands of years of human evolving, we have lived in closely knit kin relationships. In our modern industrialized world the strength of kin relationships has been broken by the slavemasters of the old smokestack industries and by the modern slavemasters of corporate giants who demand that you belong to their family, not your own.

The nuclear family has been praised and lauded, though it is the fragile, unnatural result of industrialization and loss of spiritual values. Hypocrisy within the family results from the innate fear of total aloneness. In the heyday of the flower-child movement, group marriages were tried as some people realized their need for something more than the prison of a one-on-one relationship. Open marriages have also been tried but have usually failed. These efforts were the result of the deep instinctive human need for a strong kin relationship. Forming an artificial kin group is difficult but in no way impossible, provided you share a goal, and understand that all people are not perfect.

The mutual goal of the Tantric group is the ultimate spiritual experience of Nirvana. Provided all are working toward the shared goal, many shortcomings are tolerable—though perhaps not as many as you would endure in a blood relationship. Waiting for kin with perfect form, perfect habits—waiting, that is, for perfect people—will result in nothing happening. If you will not accept those who fall short of your own arbitrarily defined perfection, that fact shows an imperfection in yourself.

The methods and life-style described herein were prevalent in the ancient world. They are based on Wiccan belief in Europe and Tantric belief in the East. These two life systems, violently suppressed when patriarchies conquered matriarchies, revered the Mother for Her life-giving powers. They also revered males for their strength and the old for their wisdom.

We cannot return to the old life-style in this modern world, but a version of it can be and has been successfully tried by a small band of dedicated students of the School of Wicca. This book results from extensive research in India and from students who have lived the system and have suggested modifications for modern practice. For these people the reward is immeasurable, in that their life has no fear or anxiety in it.

Like them, you, too, can work with dedicated purpose toward the old/new goal of becoming part of a kin, living in a Tantra house. Thus you will

- never again be alone.
- have loving, supporting friends.
- be spiritually fulfilled.
- have a purpose in life.
- achieve complete equality with the opposite gender.

The ultimate reward of Tantra is the achievement, even for a fleeting moment, of Nirvanic bliss. Inherent in Tantra is its promise of the serenity of Nirvana in months, not the years of other Yoga paths. Only in recent years has the seventh path of Ha-tha Yoga become acceptable to Vedic purists. Such reluctance may be caused by the fact that Ha-tha is a faster path to Nirvana than any of the preceding paths. Maybe some gurus have a vested interest in keeping their students around, and of course they revile the eighth path of Tantra, which is often faster than the seventh.

HOW TO USE THIS BOOK

Many believe that teaching requires gurus, but that belief became obsolete centuries ago with the invention of printing. This book will be your personal guru and will instruct you. If the instruction ever becomes difficult or painful, you have strayed from the path; for the path is full of joy and serenity.

If you don't follow the guru's instructions, the only loser is you. In that respect, the book is the perfect guru; for it has no emotional involvement with you. It is, after all, only a book. If you don't follow instructions, if you don't do things the way the guru suggests—at least the first time—who will lose? You. The book really could not care less than it cares now. It has no vanity that demands your obedience. It has no anger that will smite you if you don't follow instructions. Only you will know, and only you yourself will care if you miss the path.

Using this book requires understanding and discipline. Try to understand the development chapter by chapter, but do not slavishly follow the teaching of the guru. To gain understanding, the guru recommends you go through at least six lunar cycles of the development with at least one (and ideally more) partner(s). A group of four seems to work well as a start. Now adjust to the group's needs. Many people feel the old cleansing rituals are difficult and unnecessary; once you have given them an honest try, you may feel free to modify them. Other people like to elaborate on the rituals, making more offerings to the God-ess and fleshing out the bones the guru has given. Try the guru's path with understanding, then insert modifications and you'll progress to more perfect group rituals.

Tantra is one of the oldest pathways. The ancient texts agree that it is the quickest and easiest path to follow. Paradoxically, they also agree that in some ways it is the most difficult, because preconceived notions and trained-in ideas have to be laid aside. You have to wash away misconceptions and replace them with the clear mind on which a new philosophy can be written.

Any action can be misunderstood, misused, or made to look dirty. There are a host of words in English that people use to describe sexual behavior. Most of them have negative connotations. This says something about the way we are taught to think about sex.

In the style of Tantra described here, adult, thinking men and women work together for each other's benefit. Sex, making love, and mutual orgasms are some of the most beautiful and pleasurable things two people can do together. Whatever creator God you believe in, it must surely blaspheme Her/Him/It to deny the gifts you are given.

In the great revolt against all old religions when patriarchal sects enforced their preeminence, most Tantric scriptures were burned. The source-books, the Upanishads, the Bhagavad Gita, and the Rg Veda, still exist (though their accuracy is doubted by some). Some Tantric temples were not destroyed, so we can see in their stones the story of this great religion. In the 19th century a great revival of interest in Tantra took place. Such learned scholars as Sir John Woodruff bought and studied surviving manuscripts. The Kama Sutra was rediscovered and published at great expense in gold and pure leather as an esoteric book of high value.

Unfortunately scholars were biased by their culture. They lived in a world where women and their powers were scorned—and feared. In India today, women are still the lowest of the low. Thus the Tantra translations of those Victorian scholars were very chauvinistic and male oriented. The writers of this guru have done their best to recreate and adapt into a Western mode the ancient ideas, but the guru may in fact be inaccurate. So read and use with understanding, and feel free to make changes. Do not view it as a bible; do not imagine the guru is infallible.

If you are really to gain the greatest possible benefit from this guru, you will have to start thinking about what you do. Instead of listening to what others tell you to do, think of what they stand to gain by dominating you. Resolve to yourself: "I will no longer be dominated. From this moment on, I am my own person. Any time somebody says I must or should do something, I will ask myself, 'What do they have to gain?'"

Before you proceed to follow the guru's path, truthfully answer these simple questions: Do you really want total power and control over another human so he or she will always and instantly fulfill every sexual whim you have? Do you lust for power so that thousands will jump to your command? Do you want to be a multi-millionaire?

If you want any of these things, you should consign this guru to the fire now. If you have no control over your emotions, if you want nothing more than to copulate everlastingly or to be buried in gold, this path is not for you.

This book is written for those of you who rejoice in your body. As you learn to control it, as you learn to understand the needs of your spiritual self, so you will look behind the visible reality of another person and find the true spirit that dwells within. Tantra goes far beyond the usual pleasant but pointless sex that most humans indulge in. Sexual desires are harnessed. Other people can have irresponsible sexual relationships, and then leave each other after having reached their goal. In contrast, the goal of Tantra is to gain ecstasy beyond the physical coupling. A few have glimpsed that ecstasy through other techniques, but you should achieve it easily and surely with the aid of Tantra.

PART
ONE

BASIC PRECEPTS

CHAPTER
ONE

Roots and Definitions

IN PAKISTAN, ON the Indus River in the ancient city of Mohenjo Daro, stands a monument bearing a golden seal, reliably dated as being 6,000 years old. It depicts a person sitting in a Yoga posture performing a Tantric ritual. This is the oldest evidence known of Tantric Yoga, the Royal Path of sexual Yoga, sometimes called the eighth path. The religion of Tantra antedates both Hinduism and Buddhism. The great religion of Tantra was suppressed because it was very female oriented, but Tantra persisted in verbal tradition and in some ancient texts.

Present-day Tantrists can use translations of some very ancient texts, the foremost being the Bhagavad Gita. Many Tantric practices stem directly from verses in the Gita. Other Tantra sources are the sayings (or sutras) of Patanjali, which date from some 2,300 years ago. Thus in studying Tantra you are embarking on a path that has signposts—but also a path whose very existence is anathema to the patriarchal establishment and to present-day orthodox religions. Tantrists are despised, maligned, and put down by the new traditionalists, lest their followers depart to follow the path of Tantra.

Tantra is an extension of Ha-tha practice—an extension that uses sex and power (prana) raised from the human body. Tantrists get themselves into deep trouble with modern conventional religious philosophies, in that what a conventional religionist may label blasphemous or immoral behavior, the Tan-

trist considers moral and non-blasphemous. The Tantrist
believes that to disregard any element of human potential is to
blaspheme the handiwork of the Deity.[1]

To the Tantrist, the understanding of natural sensory pleasures comes only after experiencing the pleasure. You eat well of
delectable food, then have totally tasteless food, then fast; in
this way you gain discipline through voluntarily giving up pleasure, and enjoy the pleasure more by contrasting it with the
time of withdrawal.

Tantrists scorn the ascetic, for they say the ascetic, never
having experienced pleasure, is giving up nothing. Because sensory feelings are transient, you must alternate between experiencing sensory pleasure and withdrawing from it. Withdrawal
can last for extended lengths of time when the Tantrist goes on
the full cleansing fast; but normally the cycles run with the
moon, ranging from sensory satiation to deprivation of the
appetites within each lunar month.

Tantrists also disagree with those who take the path of pain.
They agree with the theory that pain and pleasure are indeed
opposites which must be reconciled; but they point out that the
whole aim of the work of people who endure unnecessary pain is
to suppress feelings or entrance themselves so they feel no pain.
Suppressing natural feelings rather than tuning them to a high
level of awareness is the very reverse of the Royal Path.

Your guru takes the attitude that what is natural and pleasurable is right and normal; what is unnatural is taboo. In defining the word "natural" we immediately come to the first of many
difficult decisions. The simplest way of defining "natural" is 1)
it's acceptable in your own cultural matrix; and 2) when you join
a Tantric group, it's acceptable to all members of the group
without exception. If there is any question as to whether something is natural, it may be tried but not made part of the group
rituals until all members agree about it. As you proceed along

---

[1]In this sense God is neither male nor female.

the path, you will learn to distinguish that which for your group is natural and right from that which is unnatural.

Many texts wrongly accuse Tantra students of committing unnatural acts; however, the very essence of true Tantra is that anything that should be done must be pleasurable and natural. Only the most sadistic or vicious man could possibly enjoy raping a virgin—yet we are told that this was the high point of ancient Tantra ritual. An exactly similar claim was made in the West by defamers of Wicca. Sexual pleasure is achieved with a skilled partner, not with a virgin of either gender. Since exquisite pleasure is the aim, there is absolutely no point in a Tantrist having sex with an inexperienced partner.

Similarly, Tantrists were accused of eating the most loathsome things and drinking until their senses were totally anesthetized. Neither of these practices can result in exquisite pleasure. Tantra has its prescribed eating habits which involve the eating of delectable foods properly prepared and the drinking of moderate amounts of fine wine. The palate must never be numbed by overindulgence, and Tantric exercises cannot be fully enjoyed when one is satiated with food or wine.

THE THREE PATHS

As you proceed with your study of Tantra, you will learn that its path is threefold:

1. *The mental path*, in which all things prescribed, including the exercises, are done only in the imagination. The traditional Tantrist scoffs at this path, believing it was invented as sop for those who could not do the exercises.

2. *The right-hand path*, followed by many, stipulates the exercises be done only by marriage partners working together. Again the orthodox Tantrist scorns this path on two counts: a) As everyone recognizes, the ability to do a sexual act with your spouse

does not guarantee that it results in the maximum pleasure, for having sex with a "different" partner can result in more pleasure, especially if that different partner is skilled; and b) the Tantrist has no belief in the spiritual authority of a civil marriage, holding instead that marriage is an unhealthful state forced on the general population. This civil state has no parallel in nature. The Tantrist does not in any way despise romantic love or romantic relationships; and many Tantrists form long-lasting attachments with a specific partner. But an orthodox Tantrist does not contractualize such an attachment, for it is a spiritual matter, not a civil one. A Tantrist would also point out that spiritual growth does not necessarily occur at the same rate in two partners, whether or not they are legally tied to each other, and it is a blasphemy to tie an advanced spirit to a less-developed one. A woman whose spirit is advanced must have the freedom to advance further by associating with a male of her own level.

3. *The Royal Path* – The genuine Tantrist is of the High or Royal Path. This has occasionally been called the left-hand path purely for derogatory reasons. A 20th-century Tantrist said, "We are happy to have it called the Left-Hand Path – for is not the left hand controlled by the right half of the brain? That is, the side of the brain in which all artistic enterprises dwell?" The High Path requires sexual contacts between consenting adults, within their own carefully selected and trained group.

If a married couple wishes to form their own royal group or to enter a Tantric house, they must first obtain a legal divorce and live with the divorce for at least a year and a day. Only thus can the necessary freedom from the very human emotion of jealousy be achieved.

All the warnings, all the negative stereotypes attached to Tantra, cannot efface from the ancient Sanskrit writings the fact that Nirvana is achieved more quickly through Tantra than through any other path. The scripture promises that Nirvana can be achieved in as little as six lunar months. We believe that a realistic schedule is a year – and then only if the last six months are spent in serene surroundings. It should be emphasized that once you have learned the High Path you can use from it that which you will. You can do as little of it or as much of it as you like. Do only what feels natural. If a given exercise does not feel natural to you today, you may come to it at some time in the future. If you find part of the path painful and difficult to achieve, come back to the guru; for it may be that you have strayed from the Way. The true Way is one of pleasure and happiness. There is no place for tears or sadness in Tantra.

If you find that by pursuing the path you cause great unhappiness or pain to another human being, leave the path temporarily until you can follow it without harming or causing pain to anyone. This may mean severing a relationship – but you mustn't hold back for someone you've outgrown. That constitutes self-harm, and that's no better than other-harm.

TABOOS

Throughout this book we will mention certain taboos that occur in Tantra practice. Taboos serve more as signposts that will help you pursue your path with pleasure, rather than being rigid prohibitions. You will find that when you break a taboo there will be no earth-shattering cataclysmic upheaval in your life and you won't become suddenly less spiritually aware. What will happen is that a little pain or distress will come in. This will point up the breaking of a taboo.

Let us look at one such taboo, an age taboo. It is normal that those involved in Tantra practice shall be within 15 years of one another's age. This taboo normally prohibits parent-child relationships, but it does not taboo brother-sister relationships. The brother and sister would be consenting adults and would take care to prevent conception.

Another restriction is that it is normally taboo for male hands to insert the lingam into the yoni. Insertion is to be done by female hands. This taboo precludes rape in any Tantra house.

During certain phases of the month certain activities are taboo—or as a Tantrist would say, "We accentuate certain positive activities rather than forbid others."

In today's climate of sexually transmitted diseases that can kill, there is one basic taboo. It is a prime and inviolable rule of the group that *outside* sexual contacts are forbidden and are cause for immediate, non-negotiable dismissal from the group.

In every group the taboos should be written down and understood by all members. This society is not barbaric or unthinking or uncaring. The traditional rules of the social civilized matrix from which the house members come form the basis for the rules of the house itself. The only rules that are bent are those pertaining to a government's control of the religious practices of its citizens and the rights of free, consenting adults to do as they wish in the privacy of their home.

Blatant contravention of laws designed for public welfare and order is not the Tantric way. Most especially Tantrists have no need of illegal drugs, because the path brings its own natural highs.

DEFINING THE INDEFINABLE

There has been a general move among Western writers to define in concrete mechanistic terms many ideas and concepts of Tantra—and indeed Yoga—that are really indefinable. The whole Yoga movement was done a massive disservice when inexperienced translators made various spiritual centers or chakras synonymous with specific places in the body. The spiritual body is not part of the mundane body. It coexists with it, but the chakra is in the spiritual body, not in the mundane body. The spiritual body does not have genitalia or an anus, and to define a spiritual center as coexisting with the genitalia is utter rubbish. The third eye is not the pineal gland; it is part of the spiritual body, the "I."

To understand this concept from the Tantrist's point of view, let us start by trying the impossible: to define God.

THE TANTRIST'S ULTIMATE DEITY

To a Tantrist, the Ultimate Deity cannot be defined. This non-definition has received a great deal of definition by Western writers! Whole texts have been written on the yin-yang. Some of the definitions resemble the Buddhist's Great Void or the Hindu Rama, who is the "summation of everything." Others define it as *That*, which contrasts with *This*, the plane in which we live. We cannot define the indefinable. Any definition we suggest limits the powers of an Ultimate Deity; nonetheless, philosophers will continue trying to satisfy the human longing for definition.

The Ultimate Deity is beyond mind. It has neither logic nor illogical behavior. It exists, beyond the mind and beyond thought.

Throughout this book we will refer to the Ultimate Deity as IT. Please remember, though, that such a definition is flawed; for in saying IT we think of Something which exists alone. IT both exists and does not exist. IT is infinite and finite. IT is everywhere but nowhere.

"I," "Me," and "IT"

In Tantric thought, as in many other philosophies, the personality is composed of three parts. Tantra holds that a tiny part of IT inhabits each body, being the body's spiritual component. This little piece of IT is the "I." The "I" is the real part of the person, the part that reincarnates to inhabit many shells or bodies. "I" controls two important subsidiaries: the body and the mind. In your own life you recognize this distinction, for you say "my arm," or "my leg," or "my mind." It is a basic tenet of Yoga that the mind must be as well controlled as the body. If you are angry, you may think of striking someone or smashing something. "I" controls "Me" the body, and prevents it from doing this inappropriate action.

The ancient writings offer a clear metaphor, comparing each individual to a driver and a chariot. You own your body. You run it around . . . "and the reins are Wisdom."

THE COMBINATION OF OPPOSITES

It is not possible to revere an IT, nor can you blame IT. IT is altogether beyond emotions such as vanity and anger, nor does IT care very much about you the individual and your little ego. Humans need some representation of IT, however, that we can praise, blame, pray to, and do all the other things that we need to do in reaching toward the Ultimate Deity. God-ess images are simply an interface we create in our own image with our own energies to meet our own needs.

The gods of the Hindu and Buddhist pantheons are very complex, yet easily understood if each aspect is studied singly. In this book we will deal with them as mundane conceptual God-esses. It is not a matter of knowing their names and attributes; instead it is the gaining of a comprehension of the level and thought of each God-ess in turn.

The two great gods of Tantra are Shakti (the mother goddess) and Shiva (the virile male god). These two deities are shown with many arms and many attributes. It is recognized that the female is both the giver of life and its taker-away. She can be aspected like a lover or she can be aspected like a mother, a matron, or a wise crone. In a similar way the male can be the destroyer or the creator. He can be the angry avenger or the wise old man. In Tantra he is generally the more passive, obtaining life and illumination from the female. From now on we will use the name Shakti for the Great Mother archetypal goddess and Shiva for the Great Father god.

THE MACROCOSM AND THE MICROCOSM

From time immemorial it has been held as a tenet of mystical thought that in this microcosm of ours we represent the macrocosm and the multiverse. The structure of a galaxy resembles the structure of an atom. We are cared for by our mother and father. Hence it is easy to believe in a Great Mother and Father somewhere benevolently caring for the multiverse, and beyond them an Ultimate Deity of which we cannot conceive.

We call them IT, Shakti, and Shiva. Nothing further is possible; for IT is a summation of all that is. In thinking of a poor human living his or her life on the earth plane, it is conceived that within each human the I is a piece of IT. But since each human is either male or female, only when male and female are actually joined in sexual union is there completion. For when the two are joined, we have everything that is. The combination of opposites makes the whole. If the opposites cannot be understood, and through combination wholeness cannot be experienced, then life is meaningless.

We have in the microcosm IT, Shakti, and Shiva. We have "I," the male, and the female, making a perfect miniature of the Whole. This is the meaning of the yin and the yang. When the male and the female are joined together, God-ess is forever present. Bliss can be achieved in a single human being only when the need for balancing maleness and femaleness is removed. To the Tantrist, this need is removed only when the two are joined, or at death.

The total spiritual universe is viewed as IT, plus Shakti, Shiva and life. These three levels are reflected in the microcosm of our own selves when sexual union occurs. IT as spirit is ever-present. Our bodies represent the plane of Shakti and Shiva, and the earth we rest on is the life. Thus is the macrocosm reflected in the microcosm. This state cannot be achieved while sexual lust is present; it must be controlled and put aside. This can happen only when male and female genitalia are in contact for extended periods, preferably with the lingam in the yoni. To fulfill ritual requirements perfectly, the male must maintain the erect lingam, and the female must be aroused. Because of the fragility of the erection without desire, the male is not ridiculed if the erection cannot be maintained. In fact only he and his partner will know that they did not attain the full yin-yang coalescence. Partial coalescence is attained if the partners press the lingam against the yoni while they maintain a deeply pene-trating kiss.

Traditionally such Maithunic coupling is maintained for 32 minutes and no orgasm is expected or desired by either partner. Many couples find that orgasm is an urgent necessity about an hour after completing the ritual; of course there is no ban on this completion.

Outsiders have labeled this Tantric coupling sinful or lust-ful, but Nirvana cannot be achieved when lust is present. In sacred ritual coupling, lust is absent. The concept of sin has long been used to control the actions of uninitiated people. To the Tantrist, those unenlightened people who live outside the Tan-tric discipline are not only missing part of life, but are also blaspheming IT. The codes of behavior laid down for the unini-tiated are usually politically motivated, for the Tantrist will point out, "If I am happy and content, I will not need to work any more than I do, or pay heed to other people's commands and rules. Through gaining Nirvana, I am released; and one who has not experienced Nirvana does not have the right to tell me what I should or should not do. If he thinks my deeds are wrong, he need not imitate them."

To deliberately avoid gaining Nirvana, by whatever method, is a blasphemy in the true Tantrist's mind. The Tantrist will not lay a guilt trip on someone else or on himself if he temporarily suspends his working toward Nirvana. For he knows that by laying a guilt trip on someone else he will inevitably draw that negativity to himself. "They will all come to it eventually," says the Tantrist. Nature cannot safely be denied. When natural behavior is denied, crime, pain, and war inevitably follow. The Tantrist will pursue the path with the knowledge that he or she is avoiding the blasphemy of failing to reach toward the Ultimate.

TANTRIC SPIRITUAL PROGRESS

If all Tantric ritual is healthful and contains no sin, how does the Tantrist judge his or her progress? Progress is judged by the attainment of the blissful state of Nirvana and helping others to attain such a state. Merit is achieved by perfecting the ritual, by perfecting one's behavior, by eliminating the various all-too-human emotions we fall prey to, by controlling all body functions, by helping others to understanding, and by combining and melding with opposites. When a ritual is perfected, the person who performs it is made more perfect.

This is the real basis of the old alchemical metaphor of transmuting lead into gold. Materialistic people have thought that the alchemist pursuing his dream was trying literally to transmute the metal lead into the metal gold. What he was trying to do was to convert himself from spiritual lead into spiritual gold. It matters not what we do, whether we dig a ditch, perfect a ritual, or paint a picture. The more perfectly we try to do it, the more merit we gain. By doing it perfectly, our spirit grows. Everything is in the trying. It is no loss of merit when failure occurs, and we are not discouraged from trying again; for by trying we learn. Ultimately, enough merit is accrued by a spirit so when the body it inhabits "dies," spirit recombines with IT and achieves ultimate spiritual Nirvana.

TRANSCENDING THE FEAR OF DEATH

One of the oldest beliefs of Tantra is a sure knowledge that the spiritual part, the "I," goes on to other levels when the body "dies." Very early in Indian thought the "law-giver" Manu changed the whole concept of reincarnation as a system of progressive, orderly growth and development, and replaced it with the utter chaos of transmigration. Manu understood that if people could not be threatened with a worse next-life they could not be mentally controlled and forced into religious docility in their present life. So he said, "If you are bad in this life you will come back as a loathly beast in the next life." As a control system, this closely resembles that used by various Christian sects. They outlawed the idea of reincarnation in A.D. 553; then they had to bring in a threat system called hell to keep their

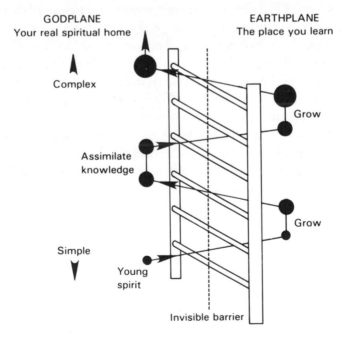

Figure 1.   Progressive reincarnation.

victims in line. "If you are bad—that is, if you violate the system of arbitrary do's and don'ts we've set up—you will burn in eternal fire."

Tantrists use the older, more natural and logical reincarnation system as the basis for much of what they do. They hold that the world is a classroom, that "I" inhabits a body in this classroom in order to develop and grow. When "I" has learned all it can from inhabiting this specific body in this specific classroom, it will go on, perhaps to inhabit other, more complex bodies in other planetary systems; or perhaps to rejoin IT.

Glance now at figure 1. It shows the progress and growth of a spirit on the earth plane. The little seed spirit, a little piece of IT, becomes the "I" of a tiny, simple living creature. When the being dies, "I" crosses the Invisible Barrier; after a time in the plane of IT,[2] "I" returns to inhabit a slightly more complex body on the physical plane.

As the "I" grows, it becomes able to control a more complex body and the problems assigned to it become more difficult to solve. Let us examine a small segment of this growth process and compare it to a child going through school. On the first day at school, a child needs to adjust to the classroom environment. Gradually the child learns the way things are done and acquires new knowledge. His or her comprehension grows. This is the microcosmic representation of the spirit coming to the classroom of life. The spirit is not evil or bad if it does something wrong; it is just undeveloped. As a child learns in school, so the spirit learns in life. The child must return to school many times before graduation. In a similar way, the spirit returns many times to inhabit earth-plane shells to learn all it must before it graduates.

Death does not necessarily mean that you are through with your lives on earth; though if you have achieved Nirvana many times through Tantra, it is likely that you will not have to return

---

[2]Describing IT as being "in a plane" is incorrect, but we know of no better way. Such words as sphere, area, place, and volume are all misleading.

to the earth plane. If, through lack of awareness, you have done something very negative, you will not be condemned to eternal fire or come back as a loathly beast. It indicates that you came undeveloped to this classroom of life and have not completed your schooling. You are not sinful or evil; instead it means you don't know the rules of the game.

The person who lays a guilt trip on you is not a great teacher but just another kindergartener trying to make it into first grade the wrong way—by treading you down and climbing on you. You should no more listen to the "guilt tripper" than you would take the advice of any other kindergartener. When you find a great spirit who knows enough to show you the path without threats, listen; for this is indeed the way into the higher grades. One way to recognize such a great spirit is by the sense of relief and recognition you feel when you hear his or her wisdom.

Reincarnation in the Tantric sense is a progressive system. You come into human form perhaps as a spirit from a higher animal. You spend several incarnations at the human level, first as male, then as female. (The female has more areas of learning available: how to bear and care for children, for example.) Eventually you are able to get off the wheel of human incarnations.

Each cycle of life is comparable to one level of development. Thus it correlates with a specific chakra. Since there are seven chakras, ranging from the lowest development at the base to the highest at the crown, if you do everything perfectly each time you incarnate to this planet, you may complete the microcosmic cycle in seven reincarnations (or fourteen, as some schools hold, believing that each stage must be completed as both male and female).

This is not to say that you might not come back again as a great whale or inhabit another body in another planetary system. It says only that you have achieved all that can be achieved within the human frame in this world. Look very carefully at that last sentence: You have achieved all you can achieve within the human frame. That does not mean that you become a multi-millionaire. It means that you can control every function and sense you were born with, and you can experience with serenity all the negative things (as well as the positive things) of this world.

When you "die" you are graduating. This is the happy time when your spirit returns to be in a plane with the Ultimate Deity. Some Tantric sects view birth as a sad time, for they think of all the things this poor little mite coming into the world must endure.

With Manu's doctrine of transmigration arose the concept of karma and karmic debt. He was not satisfied with saying that you would come back as a loathly beast the next time; he also invented the Big Ledger in the Sky wherein your every deed is recorded. The whole doctrine of karma is superfluous in Tantric belief. The thing that records your development is the thing inside you. It is "I," your spirit. By doing things perfectly, by acquiring wisdom, the spirit grows. Since the spirit is always with you, the concept of somebody keeping a separate accounting in an akashic ledger in the sky becomes laughable.

GROWING

In nature everything grows and increases until it is attacked by some force which is also growing. It is basic to Tantric belief that the spirit naturally tries to grow. It is recognized that the spirit will be stunted if it is merely taught a set of rules which it must blindly follow. From the Tantric point of view, then, for full and beauteous spiritual growth you must not just follow prescribed rules; for when you do you are inhibiting your own growth. "Thou shalt not think"? That is not growth. It is as if you are traveling along a road and your vision is fixed only on the road, forbidden to explore the countryside along the path you are traveling. When the road becomes boring, you wander off a little. Here appears a man in a black suit who whips you back onto the road. The spirit shrivels under the whip and lash of the pronouncement that you must follow the straight and narrow path.

The spirit must be allowed to wander; otherwise growth is inhibited, as surely as if a boulder were placed on a tender seedling.

When a group is attempting a difficult task, instant and unquestioning obedience must temporarily be accorded to the leader; for without it the goal could not be achieved. If a specified goal is not achieved, change the rules and, if necessary, the leader. However, perpetual, instant and unquestioning obedience to arbitrary rules can never be justified, especially when rules are made by a power group intending to control the female half of the population and all younger males.

THE TOOLS OF TANTRA

In most chapters you will be shown practical exercises to try. To learn true Tantra and to understand the meaning of its Nirvanic bliss, it is important to practice the exercises until they become habitual, even automatic. The basic tools of Tantra that are most neglected in our Western civilization are the lingam and the yoni. To succeed in Tantra, these two essential tools must be exercised and brought to peak performance.

The Lingam: It is important that an erection can be obtained at will and can be maintained. Most young men get an erection at the slightest thought of sex; for them a Playboy centerfold is an adequate aphrodisiac. In later life that ease of erection is lost. The male must remember how to do it, and the erecting muscles must be exercised. The basic and most simple exercise is done early in the morning, immediately after washing and just before the sunrise ritual. The male stands in the erecting position (figure 2) and, just by willing it, gains an erection. If he cannot at first obtain the erection by willing it, the female may help by gently massaging the lingam. An erection firm enough to support a hand towel (approximately four ounces) is required. As confidence and skill are gained, the male learns to relax the first erection and then re-acquire it. Bathing the lingam in cold water will often achieve this relaxation for the inexperienced male. Each new erection must be sufficiently strong to hold a hand towel. Four erections are usually done for a complete exercise cycle.

Some students find that when they first attempt this it can be done with relative ease, but that it becomes more difficult as the level of interest falls with the passage of time. They should

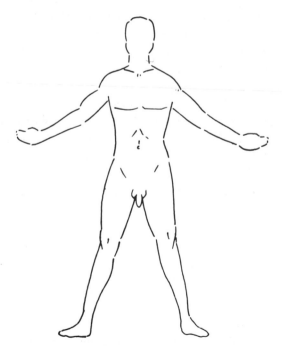

Figure 2. Erecting position.

remember that they are extending their sexual life by many years through this simple exercise, for with its repetition the erectile muscles maintain good tone and condition.

The Yoni: In Western culture yonic exercises are almost unknown. They are regarded as something to be snickered about in the bathroom. For good, healthful, long-lasting sexual activity, however, the yonic muscles must be properly exercised. Perform the first exercise in a tub of warm clean water after the shower. Lie back with the feet on the edges of the bathtub; relax the muscles totally so water can enter the yoni. Then contract the muscles strongly to force the water out with a noticeable spurt. Four such relaxations and contractions are recommended daily for the practicing female student.[3]

The group may invent many amusing exercises for each other. Suspending weights from a ring on the end of the erect lingam, the winner supporting the most weight, is perhaps matched only by how tight the yogin can grip a candle so that weights can be suspended from it for a similarly harmless and entertaining competition.

Another Tantric ritual often misunderstood is the adoration of the lingam and the yoni and their anointing with natural oils. When stripped down to its essence, what is happening is a ritualistic lubrication of the parts, which sometimes become chafed. To lubricate the lingam, olive oil is gently massaged in, together nowadays with oils that contain lanolin. Of course the massaging is done by a female. In a similar way the lubrication of the yoni is enhanced by the application of glycerin and lanolin. This internal application is gently done by the male. Lightly scented oil is often used: patchouli for the male and musk for the female.

---

[3]Once the yogin has learned to expel water, she can do the exercise while she lies on her back on an exercise mat. These contractions have recently been rediscovered in the West, where they are called Kiegel contractions.

SUNRISE RITUAL

Every morning as the sun appears over the horizon, the following ritual is done by all initiated members of the household.[+]

All the members of the household arise. After relieving their bodies of waste material, they wash face, hands, and genitalia with cool water and unscented soap. No one speaks. The male lies on the exercise mat with his hands toward the sun. The female takes the astride position with the lingam vitae completely encased in the yoni. The male parts his knees and places the flat soles of his feet together; he places his hands above his head with the palms together. In this position, the soles of the female's feet are under his thighs. She spreads her arms wide with palms upward. She tips her head slightly backward and lifts her breasts with her pectoral muscles. The male positions his hands so the palms rest lightly under her breasts, then replaces his hands above his head. They both take two full, deep breaths. The female firmly contracts her yoni eight times in slow succession. In time with her the male enlarges his lingam. With her right hand, the yogin welcomes the sun by touching in turn the four chakras near the brow, the throat, the heart, the genitalia. As she does this she says, "Father, I understand the health the sun will bring me. Bless you for growing the food I will eat today. Let my heart send strength through my body to do your will. Beloved Mother of all, be happy that the earth receives the sun."

She leans down and rests her forehead on the male's forehead. To help this, he places his hands behind his neck and lifts his head. In unison they speak the first words: "Mother to Father, Father to Mother, all is well. Good morning."

The female dismounts. If there are an equal number of males and females, she lies in the nesting position (the opposite side of the male from which she usually sleeps with him). If there

---

[+]The ritual is also allowed to pre-initiates (candidates) at the option of the elders of the house.

is a gender imbalance in the house the "extra" males or females repeat the ritual with other partners. Then all snuggle together. It is true, of course, that after nesting for some time the yogi and yogin may make love. There is no reason why they should not, provided that after the ritual they observe a nesting of eight minutes before sexual activity commences.

It is important to Tantrists that each lingam be encased in a yoni at or near the rising of the sun, and that each yoni be penetrated at the same time. Nobody gets left out. A yogin who is menstruating does the same rite, but the lingam is gently brought forward onto her lower abdomen instead of being encased in the yoni. The rite is very sacred and is not open to outsiders or observers.

The care of your Tantric tools, the lingam and the yoni, is your sacred duty. As people forget to exercise and as they age, they tend to let the various sexual and other muscles go flabby. Tantra teaches that the muscles must be exercised and must be controlled. Gaining an erection is not a psychological matter; it is just a matter of muscular control. A flabby lingam or yoni is an unhealthy one. When these muscles are in good condition, the rest of the body also functions in a more healthy way. Gradually through this book we will introduce you to other exercises you should practice to improve the whole body tone. In Tantra you learn that enough is enough. We are not trying to become athletes or to develop bulging muscles. To be vibrantly healthy is enough.

CONTRACEPTION

In all Tantra practice the responsibility for contraception lies with the yogin. If the yogi has had a vasectomy, he should obviously tell those in the house that he is infertile. The whole decision about when or whether to conceive and whom to conceive with rests squarely on the shoulders of the yogin. It is her right — no, it is her duty — to conceive only in a responsible way.

She alone makes all decisions about her own reproductive system and whether or not she wishes to have children. She must judge her suitability from the point of view of her family's genetic history and decide about reproducing with this and other factors in mind. In Tantra the fetus has no spirit until it has been born and taken eight breaths. Until then, it amounts to a growth on the uterus and may be aborted at the yogin's decision.

Pregnancy is welcomed with joy in any Tantra house, and the pregnant yogin is cherished and honored in every possible way. She has only light duties and is altogether in a state of bliss. She is watched and guarded and in many ways treated as an honored guest; for the signs of fecundity which she exhibits are held in high esteem.

The yogin normally has at least three yogis from whom she can choose as the donor of sperm. To avoid internal friction in the house, she usually gives no indication about which one she has selected. The first rule must be that she selects someone who has no known genetic problems; for obviously she does not wish her child to have any hereditary defects such as diabetes, Tay-Sachs disease, or any other of some 3,000 known inheritable diseases. A history of any such disease in a yogi's family should automatically disqualify him as a sperm donor. The yogin will then select on the basis of stature, choosing someone whose physical size is similar to her own. She may select someone slightly larger; but a great mismatch is to be avoided if she is to bear the child easily.

Throughout this chapter we have emphasized that natural behavior is all-important. Some may quibble that the yogin's "cold-blooded" selection of a sperm donor is not "natural." On the contrary: In Tantric thought it is the most natural of behaviors for the yogin to elect to have a healthy, happy baby. In the wild, male vertebrates go through elaborate, even ruthless, selection processes to ensure that only the fittest beget. Animal mothers instinctively select the fittest "alpha" male to beget their offspring. Can an intelligent, thoughtful yogin do less?

CHAPTER

TWO

Raising the Force

IN DIFFERENT TIMES and different cultures many names have been given to the Third Power. Nowadays we simply call it "the force." This term, popularized by George Lucas in *Star Wars*, seems to be readily understood and accepted.

The force is not the potential power of a physical object when it falls; nor is it the force of motion. Instead it is a subtle power that Tantrists call prana. Every living thing contains this latent power. In old Tantric practice the power was often called the "Shakti power" or the "raising of kundalini," for Tantrists observed that it is often associated with being sexually "turned on." When the "serpent is raised," the force is available.

The force is raised from your own body. In this chapter and its exercises you will learn to feel it, to maximize your output of it, and to tune it. Since earliest times the goal of Tantrists has been the development of the individual's highest potential. Your potential will be realized through learning to use your own body and mind.

The human body, naked and unadorned, is the highest and most beautiful form of the natural selection process that has yet been attained on this planet. To adorn it, to paint it, to perfume it, are blasphemous actions. Within many Tantric houses, therefore, nudity is the general rule if the weather permits it. When you are nude without jewelry or body paint, you are "heaven-clad." In the atmosphere of mutual trust and relaxed experimen-

tation that prevails in such a house, manifestations of the force
are easily observed. Many Westerners scoff at the idea of such a
force. They bind their tense bodies in tight clothing and wear all
sorts of jewelry. In these circumstances, it is little wonder the
force is so difficult to observe.

Many women naturally exhibit innate powers. It is an absolute fact that Muslim males made their women wear finger-rings
so that the power would be inhibited, and that Christian cru-
saders, seeing the subservience of Muslim women to their mates,
brought the idea of the wedding ring back to Europe. Nowadays
watch straps, class rings, and wedding rings adorn human
hands. All of these hinder the manifestation of the force. Of
course, rings are not worn in a Tantric house.

FEELING THE FORCE

Hold up your left hand as shown in figure 3, and point the
fingers of your right hand toward the palm of your left.[1] Keep
the fingertips about one inch from the secondary palm. Now
slowly move the forearm up and down so the fingertips pass
(without touching) across the palm of the secondary hand, as
the vertical arrows (figure 3) show. You should feel a kind of
breeze or lightness or tingling as the fingers move vertically past
the palm. That is the force, prana, the energy field that shows
up in Kirlian photography. It is the energy that you can learn to
send out to influence other human beings. Russian scientists
have shown that it can be detected at distances of 3,000 miles.

---

[1]This assumes you are right-handed. If you are left-handed, reverse the hands
in this test and put out the energy from your left hand as it points at the palm
of your right hand. If you are right-handed, your right hand is dominant; if
you are left-handed, the reverse is true. From your dominant hand flows the
energy that makes things happen. You use your secondary hand as a receiver
of energy and to psychometrize objects. This technique prevents you impress-
ing your own emotions on the object you are trying to read.

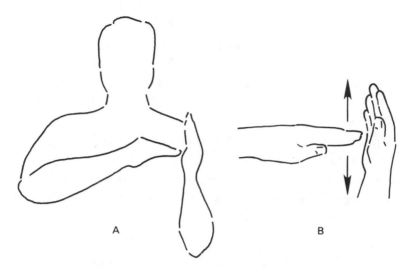

Figure 3. Hands across palm.

At this stage of your development, the experiment may not feel terribly successful to you; but practice and the knowledge contained in this chapter will teach you to feel and to use the force more readily.

The intensity of the sensation varies. Sometimes when you try to demonstrate the energy field to a friend, he or she may or may not be able to detect it. This happens because the power output varies with four major influences of your life:

1) the phase of the moon; 2) sexual influences; 3) the food you eat; 4) the time of day.

At the School of Wicca in 1972 we started testing students for these influences. We found that:

1) The energy was at maximum three to four days after the full moon and three to four days after new moon. This means that the energy relates to the tidal flow of the oceans, which also

shows the same three-day hysteresis effect. It also tends to maximize one hour after sunrise and one hour after sunset.

2) The energy is maximized when two people of opposite gender are involved. It comes to a peak about one hour after coition is interrupted, provided there is a real expectation of completion in the near future; in other words, both partners are exquisitely turned on.

3) The energy is maximized at the end of a fast, just before a heavy meal is anticipated.

4) The energy is maximized one to two hours after awakening from sleep. In general between 9 and 10 A.M. was highest in standard "first-shift" lifestyle.

If you want to test these results yourself, try the hands-across-palm at various times of the day. Fill in Table 1 based on the following instructions. Conduct the hands-across-palm experiment at the hours shown in the left-hand column of Table 1. Enter a check mark in the appropriate weak/average/strong

Table 1. Maximizing Your Force

Hour of Day	Weak			Average			Strong		
	1	2	3	1	2	3	1	2	3
1 A.M.									
3 A.M.									
5 A.M.									
7 A.M.									
9 A.M.									
11 A.M.									
1 P.M.									
3 P.M.									
5 P.M.									
7 P.M.									
9 P.M.									
11 P.M.									

column. Each Column 1 should be used on a day when you have abstained from orgasm for three days. Each Column 2 should be used just before orgasm. Each Column 3 is meant to be used a few minutes after orgasm. Take at least thirty days to complete the table.

Experiment 1: Feeling the Force

Stand face to face with a partner of the opposite gender. Hold your right hand palm up and your left hand palm down. Have your partner do the same thing. Arrange your hands as in figure 4a on page 30, so your fingers are parallel but the hands are not touching. As you stand there, in the space between the palms, energy and heat will gradually build up for about a minute and then level off. Now have your partner put his or her secondary hand vertical. Use your dominant hand to do the fingers-across-palm experiment while you maintain the other hands (your secondary hand and your partner's dominant hand) with fingers parallel and a small separation between the hands. A very intense sensation is usually felt in the palm of the receiving student. To experience this sensation yourself, reverse the positions so that you're the receiver and your partner is the transmitter. Figure 4b on page 30 shows this. To switch off the flow of power, change the non-working hands from a fingers-parallel position to a position in which the fingers of the two hands are at right angles to each other (figure 4c on page 30). It is as if you switched off a light bulb—the flow instantly ceases.

If you have a partner, at the same time on successive days, try the following experiments while abstaining from orgasms. If you do not have a partner, use any means you know will work to turn yourself on sexually. (In Tantra masturbation is not held to be evil or harmful.) With gays of various genders and various sexual preferences, we have found that this experiment sometimes works and sometimes doesn't. It seems that some gays

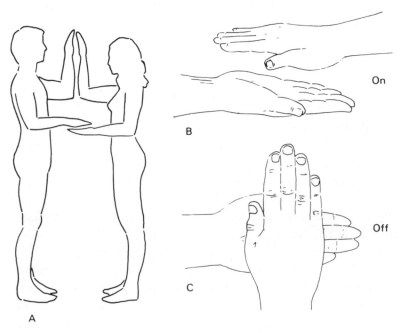

Figure 4.   Detection of cross-gender force.

have a male spirit in a female body or a female spirit in a male body. If a gay of this type works with a "straight," or with a gay of the opposite spiritual gender, the experiment works, generating about the same amount of power as it does with two heterosexuals of unlike gender. However, some gays who apparently are male spirits in male bodies or female spirits in female bodies have no success with the experiment. It is therefore best for gays to try it with several different partners and gauge from empirical results what works best. There is no guilt or blame attached to any of these experiments; they simply illustrate the laws of physics in action.

Experiment 2: Force Variations

Day 1: Do the experiment shown in figure 4. Then hug and kiss your partner until both of you are sexually aroused. Repeat the experiment. Bring the lingam into contact with the yoni. Back off, and repeat the experiment. Allow the lingam to enter the yoni and make some motion. When you are both close to orgasm, back off and repeat the experiment.

Day 2: Repeat Day 1.

Day 3: Repeat Day 1, except at the conclusion both partners come to orgasm and repeat the hands-across-palm experiment 10 minutes after orgasm.

Typical results are shown in figure 5. Of course, these results are very subjective and no arbitrary scale can be used. Figure 5 summarizes work done by hundreds of our students.

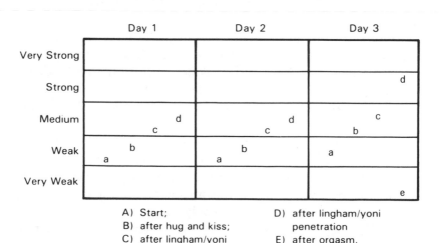

A) Start;
B) after hug and kiss;
C) after lingham/yoni contact;
D) after lingham/yoni penetration
E) after orgasm.

Figure 5.   Standard variations in force.

The sudden and dramatic drop in power after orgasm has led to an unusual sect of Tantrists who believe it is the loss of seminal fluid and the absorption of its maleness by the female that causes the death of the force. They believe that each "little death" brings death closer; so at the moment of ejaculation they either physically close off the base of the lingam and force the seminal fluid into the bladder, or use muscle control to suck the fluid into the bladder. These men train themselves by placing the lingam mortis into a glass of water and learning the "elephant trick" of drawing water into themselves. Most other Tantrists, both ancient and modern, believe that the little death is caused not by the loss of fluid but by mental activity. This is considered beneficial, so they concentrate on delaying orgasm in the mind.

As a result of your experimental work, you now know how to turn on your own force. It's fun to develop your powers by doing these experiments on a regular basis. You know how to ride the path; now learn to ride it well.

DEMONSTRATION OF THE FORCE

The easiest physical demonstration of the force is telepathic control of another person. You are sitting in a theater, waiting for the movie to start. Either alone or with another student, choose a person sitting in front of you who is not engaged in other pursuits but who, like you, is waiting passively for the movie to start. Project the force toward that person. With a little practice you can make that person turn around and look at you. In your early attempts, the target person may only scratch the back of his or her head as he or she feels a little tickle; eventually you will be able to make the person turn around on every attempt because the energy is easily felt.

The next experiment uses the children's toy called a Crookes Radiometer. Professor Crookes was a very early member of the British Psychical Research Society; he developed the radiometer to demonstrate the force. The radiometer revolves when exposed to light. Arrange it so it turns very slowly when a flashlight is shone at its blades. By directing the force at the radiometer, you can make it speed up and slow down. It is particularly impressive if two students of opposite genders do this, one holding the palm behind the radiometer and the other directing the force from the fingertips through the radiometer to the palm.

Another way of demonstrating the force for your own satisfaction is to move a table-tennis ball across a clean glass tabletop. If you hold your hand cupped slightly above the ball and point your fingertips at the palm through the side of the ball on the table, you can make the ball move across the table surface. The old experimental literature notes cases in which the ball levitates slightly and tends to bounce across the surface.

You should be aware that experiments of these types work only once or twice at a session. Demonstrations of the force to yourself also fail after the first few attempts satisfy you that it is real. It is simply a matter of the mind growing tired of playing games; and the force is, after all, not something to play games with.

Experiment 3: Psychic Energy Is All Around You

This planet is unceasingly bombarded with light from the sun and with reflected light from the moon. It is also bombarded with invisible radiation that you can use in your daily life. Stand facing East, as shown in figure 6 on page 34. Hold your head slightly back and your arms extended with your right palm up and your left palm down. Wait for a moment while you feel the energy flow into your upturned palm and out from your down-turned palm. Now quickly turn each hand over so that your left palm faces upward and your right palm downward. Can you feel the change? Do it again; this time more quickly. Some skeptics may claim you are feeling nothing more than a temperature difference of the blood in your palms, but you can prove them wrong by turning your hands quickly. If you did indeed feel only

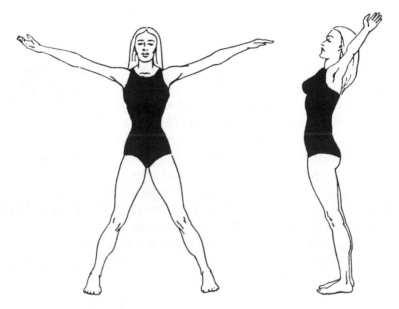

Figure 6.   Star position.

a simple temperature difference, it could not occur instantaneously — as the feeling of flowing energy does.

Every Christian agrees that of all the religious festivals, the most uplifting is the Easter sunrise service. Almost anyone you ask about such a service will tell you how inspiring it was. What did the priest or minister say? He can't tell you. What hymns were sung? He doesn't remember. What then inspired him so? Could it be that just by uplifting his hands to the sun he let into his body a tremendous burst of energy? And that this energy gave him enough of a high to sustain him for several weeks afterward? Tantrists believe very firmly that this is precisely what happened, and that the recharging procedure is a natural and necessary part of life. Such a procedure is embodied in the Tantric sunrise ritual.

Experiment 4: Sunrise Ritual

Now that you can feel and demonstrate your own force, try using it during a sunrise ritual. It gives more understanding of the reason for the sunrise ritual, which is a recharging of the yogi and the yogin. When the yogin stretches her hands outward with her palms upward, and the yogi places his palms gently under her breasts, if he maintains his feet with soles parallel and very slightly apart, he feels force flow down from her into his genitalia. The force flows to his feet where it produces a hot tickling sensation between the soles. The yogin also feels a slight warming of her breasts where his palms almost touch her. Often the nipples suddenly become hard and erect and the aureole generates intense heat.

After the sunrise greeting, when the yogin leans forward and puts her hands on the yogi's chest, he feels a definite heating and burning sensation flowing from her hands into his chest. This is a sure sign that the ritual has been completed correctly and that each partner is recharging the other. Sometimes this sensation is accompanied by a reddening of the skin under the yogin's hands, another sure sign of the force.

EARTH FORCE

Various names are given by Tantrists to the force available to them from the earth itself. From an analysis of the locations of old Tantric shrines, it is obvious that they knew the rules of what the Chinese call Feng Shui and the sorcerer calls geomancy, or earth force.

At certain places in the world it is easier to get psychically charged or turned on. At these sites you can pick up energies

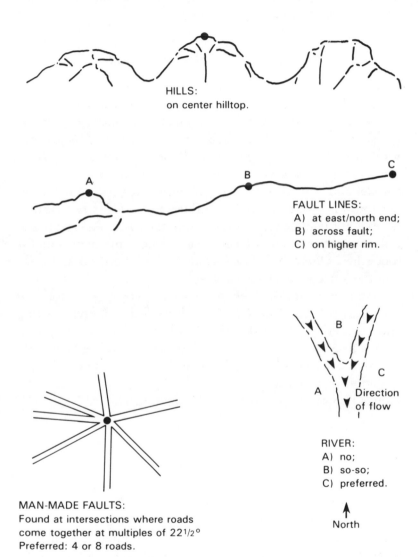

HILLS:
on center hilltop.

FAULT LINES:
A) at east/north end;
B) across fault;
C) on higher rim.

RIVER:
A) no;
B) so-so;
C) preferred.

Direction
of flow

North

MAN-MADE FAULTS:
Found at intersections where roads
come together at multiples of 22½°
Preferred: 4 or 8 roads.

Figure 7.   Places of power for geomantic charging.

radiated to or from the earth (see figure 7 on page 36). Faults, certain areas near rivers, and peaks of special hills or mountains are known to Tantrists as power places.

Faults: Many of the world's great population centers are located at or near faults. The New York–Washington, DC, megalopolis and the bustling state of California both run along major fault lines. People instinctively gravitate toward geological fault lines because they feel more energetic near them.

Man-Made Faults: In the Orient the production of artificial faults is an art form. To produce artificial lines, the ancients mapped the known world and drew lines along many of the earth power lines. Along these lines they placed markers made of foreign stone: five per mile; and every 2.72 miles they placed a major ceremonial site. Places where these "ley lines" intersect are points of phenomenal power.

Rivers: One side of a river affects you in a peaceful way, while the other side energizes you so you can be more productive. Facing upstream, you are better off to charge yourself on the right bank of the flowing water and to live on the left bank. The character of a city like St. Louis demonstrates this principle. The Missouri River flows southward. The heaviest residential areas are west of the river (on the left side), while the eastern or right side is known for its industrial nature. As every reader of romances knows, the Left Bank of Paris is popularly considered a desirable place to live.

Hills: The Great Wise Guru sits on the very top of the mountain, just waiting to hand pearls of wisdom to the pilgrim who is brave and sturdy enough to scale the heights. Tops of hills and mountains are power points well known to the Tantrist. The three-hills analogy of Native American mythos demonstrates this same principle; that is, a hill equidistant between two other hills is a power center. In ancient times, the Chinese literally built a hill upon which to situate their city of Beijing. The roof of an apartment building between two other apartments is an

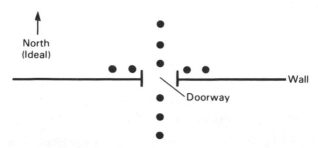

Figure 8. An artificial fault line. Each ● represents foreign stones, weighing a minimum of 5 lbs. each, spaced at intervals of 2.72 feet.

excellent charging point, as is the central hill of any mountain range.

Figure 7 shows areas that are best for getting charged up. Geological faults, rivers, mountaintops are all sources of energy. When you want to gain bounteous energy, you may live near or travel to these sites to gather a little of the energy that is available for the taking. Perhaps you live in an ordinary house or an apartment. How can you find or manufacture a point within your own physical environment so you can tap into the geomantic energy?

The simple answer is: Any discontinuity will serve. Witches have traditionally worked at the intersections of roads. Each road constitutes a man-made geological fault. House or apartment walls are also artificial fault lines. Find a wall in your home that runs on a true East-West line. Beginning at a doorway in the wall, place foreign stones at intervals of 2.72 feet (32–9/16 inches) along the wall. (See figure 8.) Use the center of the doorway as your charging point. If no wall in your dwelling runs truly East-West, do the best you can.

THE FORCE FROM ABOVE

The force flows to the earth from above, from the sun, the moon, and the cosmos itself. If you are on a mountaintop, the force reaches you first and flows through you to the earth. It also flows along faults (both natural and artificial) and along rivers to re-enter the earth in the ocean or at well-known fault shrines. The characteristics of the force you receive are determined by its source, or by the position of the sun and moon (earth's major radiating and gravitational bodies) relative to you.

The source of the force is at the outermost limits of the universe. It is the background radiation that has been present since time began. Sunrise and sunset are times when the greatest amounts of force are available, and midday and midnight the least. Apparently the position of the sun overhead or under your feet affects the amount of force available.

Figure 9 shows the position of the moon relative to the sun at full and new moon. When the moon is new, it is on the same side of the earth as the sun is, and is said to be in conjunction. When the moon is full (or in opposition) it is on the opposite side of the earth from the sun. Everyone knows how important the moon's influence is on human behavior. The Tantrist uses that influence to his or her advantage.

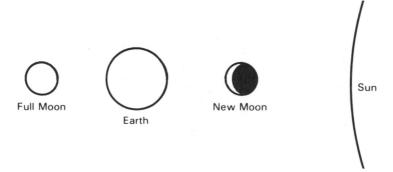

Figure 9.   Motion of the Moon relative to the Sun.

INTERACTION WITH THE FORCE

In this work so far, we have talked in terms of recharging yourself and your partner so you can turn on your force more reliably and with greater power. If you have a Tantric group with
whom to work, you can increase the force for the entire membership. All members stand in a circle, facing inward, and hold
palms slightly apart with fingers parallel. The maximum amount
of force is generated when males stand between females and
females stand between males, and all "have the serpent raised,"
or are sexually excited.

A repetitive chant which builds volume in a crescendo will
get the force flowing around the circle. At the peak of the chant,
a chosen person breaks the circle and sends the force out explo-
sively to do the will of the participants. The force here has been
stored by the people who have all recharged themselves, and is
now sent out.

Another way to build force is to use your power combined
with your partner's to control the cosmic force that flows to
earth through the area where you are working. Every living
creature has its own force field, and the earth has its own gigan-
tic force field. Tantrists believe that through correct use of your
individual force, you can become the switch that controls the

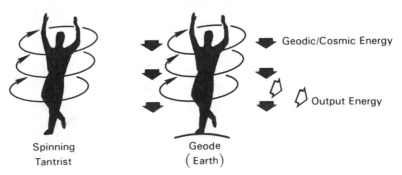

Figure 10.   The human/Earth interaction.

mighty force of the cosmos. To do this, you need to produce a rhythmic physical effort building to a peak and releasing in a sudden dumping impact. Many of you will have heard of whirling dervishes. They spin each on their own axis; or a pair spins about a common point while holding hands. When you move this way, you act like a little magnetic coil in the cosmic/earth magnetic field, as figure 10 illustrates. This spinning technique is known as the Human Earth Dynamo Effect, or HEDE. The idea is that you direct and modulate some of the earth/cosmic forces with your power.

To build up a field for positive, increasing results, you spin clockwise (in the northern hemisphere), or as Native American say, sunwise. You spin counterclockwise to generate reducing energy. This can be useful in circumstances when you want to do reducing magic, such as the elimination of a tumor.

TYPES OF FORCE

Every farmer knows that you plant downward-growing root crops when the moon is waning and upward-growing grain crops when the moon is waxing. The Tantric calendar runs four days later than the moon cycle calendar. This difference tunes it in to nature; for the tides of the ocean also run four days behind the moon's actual position.

The influence of the moon varies from day to day during the month. For now, remember that new beginnings are appropriate at the new moon and that Tantrists reach toward Nirvana at the full moon. Full moon is the time of accidents, and little or no work is undertaken during this phase. It has been found through countless experiments that certain activities are best worked on with the force at certain of the moon's phases. For every intent, a specific day of the moon's cycle is appropriate.

Each pair of the eleven-plus days between new and full moon, and between full and new moon, is assigned to one of the

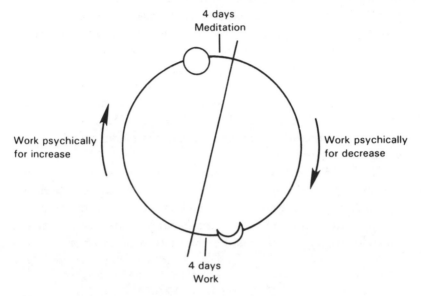

Figure 11.   The Moon cycle.

seven chakras. When Tantric work is done to increase anything:
money, love, etc., it is done on the days of the moon's increase—
when the moon is waxing. When you want to reduce anything,
you work as the moon decreases—as it wanes. (See figure 11.)
This is the same tuning of the energy that occurs when you spin
clockwise or anticlockwise in the earth's field.

TANTRA RELIANCE ON SELF

Practitioners of Western magic (sorcerers) use many outside
sources of force, such as minerals, hearth gods, pyramids, and
colored lights, to aid in their work. Tantrists, in contrast, rely
entirely on the energy available from themselves, from the
earth, and from the cosmos; for in time of urgent necessity you
may not have available all the external trappings you need.

Neophyte Tantrists may use any aid they desire; but as they gain the skills of single-pointed concentration and visualization, they are able to leave such aids behind. In some ways Tantra is a more challenging path; for the exotic mineral, the multicolored candles, and the other trappings are rarely present. The Tantrist summons the very essence of the aids into his or her single-pointed gaze and from the creative reality gains more power than if the mundane aid had been present.

Let's say Aunt Maude is ill with liver trouble. You could raise energy of a loving nature and send it to her. Will it cure her liver? Most probably not; at best it might turn her on. You sent love—but instead of sending "love," it is more appropriate to send the thought: "Cure Aunt Maude's liver!" This requires that you tune your thoughts to Aunt Maude, to her liver, and to the energy that will help cure it.

Tantrists don't know any more than physicians do why this type of psychic healing works.[2] What they do know is this: When the energy is sent out "tuned" to the problem and at the right point in the moon cycle, the results are spectacularly better than they would have been otherwise.

Over ages of experimentation, each chakra (and consequently each day of the moon cycle) has been assigned the cure of specific diseases or problems. Table 2 on page 44 shows the attributes of each chakra and the point in the moon cycle when it is best used for increase or decrease. On the appropriate day, Tantrists tune in to the attributes of the appropriate chakra before they send the force to do their bidding, through mental one-pointed visualization of the chakra and its attributes.

Western occultists add to this the correct hour and minute for the work. Tantrists know that in cases of healing it is best to do the work when a) the force can be raised to a peak; and b) the patient is receptive (which usually means asleep).

As your psychic powers develop and as you learn to use them and perhaps accomplish some psychic tasks, you will expe-

---

[2]We believe the patient's mind is influenced telepathically to cure the body.

Table 2. Rectified Table of Chakra Correspondences and Uses

Day[1]	Chakra	Element	Color	Sigil	Description
4–5	Base	Earth	Angry Red	□	Square
6–7	Pelvis	Water	Vermilion	☽	Moon
8–9	Navel	Fire	Greenish-Blue	△	Up Triangle
10–11	Heart	Air	Purple	⊗	Hexagram
12–13	Throat	Earth	Light Yellow	○	Circle
14–15	Brow	Water	Brilliant White	⋊⋉	Gate/Lingam
16–17	Crown	Fire	Light	⌇	Cup Holding
18	–	Ethers	All	⌣	–
19–20	Crown	Fire	Light	⚘	Cup Emptying
21–22	Brow	Water	White	✾	Flowering Tree
23–24	Throat	Earth	Ivory	●	Crescent Down
25–26	Heart	Air	Smoky Blue	◗	Flame
27–28	Navel	Fire	Gray	⚜	Swastika
29–30	Pelvis	Water	Dirty White	☾	Old Moon
31–32	Base	Earth	Faded Red	❖	Four Petals

Table 2. Continued

Day[1]	Chakra	Sound	Material	Animal	Usage
4–5	Base	Dark Drumming	Sulphur	Berserk Elephant	Fulfill Lust
6–7	Pelvis	Angry Sea	Salt	Hungry Crocodile	Increase Love
8–9	Navel	Thunder	Copper	Rampant Ram	Heal Genitalia & Below
10–11	Heart	Small Bells	Sapphire	Running Antelope	Improve Telepathy & the Force
12–13	Throat	Flute Upscale	Silver	White Elephant	Gain Friends
14–15	Brow	Rustling Bells	Water	Man and Woman	Heal Broken Bodies
16–17	Crown	Hot Air Rising	Space	Lotus	Heal Broken Spirits
18	–	–	Void	–	Achieve Nirvana
19–20	Crown	Smoke Rising	Space	Lotus	Reduce Spiritual Uncertainty
21–22	Brow	Rustling Chains	Water	Man and Woman	Release in Death
23–24	Throat	Flute Downscale	Ivory	White Elephant	Cure Flu, Colds, Pneumonia, etc.
25–26	Heart	Muffled Bells	Ruby	Antelope	Secure Protection
27–28	Navel	Distant Thunder	Red Gold	Ram Being Ridden	Reduce Tumors
29–30	Pelvis	Sea After Storm	Salt	Crocodile Asleep	Undergo Abortion
31–32	Base	Distant Drums	Sulphur	Working Elephant	Eliminate Enemy

[1]Moon age days after new. To stay in synch, every so often add one day of rest at full moon. The first day given is always preferred: even days for increase, odd days for decrease.

rience a sense of well-being that is impossible to gain in any other way. What seems to happen is this: As you develop and use the force your psychic body is strengthened; and when the psychic body is strengthened the physical body is strengthened with it. This is one of the reasons for Tantra's heavy emphasis on raising the force.

The force can accomplish many things: healings, the bringing of wealth, the control of other living beings and of some inanimate objects. The more selfless things you do with your developed force, the higher will you climb the ladder of the chakras toward Nirvana.

THE ETHICS OF USING THE FORCE

In Western Witchcraft a very simple ethic pertaining to the use of the force has grown up. It is summarized in the idea that you may use the force only if it does not infringe on any other person's psychic or physical space. The phrase that summarizes this is called the Wiccan Rede.

> Eight words the Wiccan Rede fulfill:
> If it harm none, do what you will.

The "none" in this instance also includes yourself. It seems to the guru that this can also be used for Tantrists. In Tantra "none" does not necessarily include beings of lower development stature. Thus in Tantra it is approved behavior for you to destroy an influenza germ to cure the human body. In some houses this is not approved, and the force may be used only when no infringement of any living creature's psyche or physical body is involved.

Tantrists use their God-given gifts to develop and to improve themselves as well as the world around them. Many people go out on crusades to improve the environment, to work with exceptional children, and to do many other things. The

Tantrist thinks this is just an externalizing of internal dissatisfaction and shortcomings. The most important thing to improve is yourself. When you yourself are perfect, THEN you can go out on your crusade and by your example can improve the world around you. In one of its wiser pages, the Judaeo-Christian Bible says, "Cast the mote out of your own eye before you try to cast the one out of your brother's" (Matt. VII:3). This is the same basic philosophy Tantrist profess. Tantrists do not try to perfect themselves completely before using their talents, however, because the use of the force in and of itself improves the practitioner.

It is also very important to Tantrists not to neglect any of the God-ess' gifts when improving yourself. Many people nowadays are out jogging and running and doing aerobic exercises and a thousand other things with which they hope to improve their muscles. These people totally neglect the improvement of their psyches and the development of their personal force. Without development of the psyche, you are incomplete.

A Word of Caution

Have fun—but don't flit blithely around showing other people all the things you can do. They will become frightened of you, and because of their fear they will attack you in any way they can. We very rarely demonstrate our powers to anyone, and we suggest you follow our example. Yes, we will do a healing, for that is something everyone pretty well accepts; but we will not make a pendulum swing or a candle go out just at the whim of anyone who asks. It is enough to know you can do it yourself.

CHAPTER
THREE

Expanding Your Awareness

ONE PURPOSE OF Tantra is the development of your own psychic powers and awareness. This guru assumes that you have a small group to help you and that there are some dyadic couples who can work together. The mode of awareness presently dominant in you may be classified into one or more of the following categories:

Clairvoyance: If your awareness is in this category, visual images and pictorial impressions are your strongest way of understanding the world around you and of getting information psychically.

Clairaudience: A much smaller proportion of people rely on their hearing for their awareness. This is obviously true of blind people in experiencing everyday life, but some sighted people are so attuned to music and noises that their awareness works through the sense of hearing. They "hear the sound" of a person who approaches them. They "hear voices" telling them things.

Clairtactition: These people experience the world through their sense of touch. When a psychic experience comes to them, the sensitive areas of their fingertips "feel" by such simple changes as feeling hot or cold, rough or smooth.

Clairtastition: The expression, "He leaves a bad taste in my mouth," comes from this form of awareness. The taste buds are able to sense minute differences in stimuli. The taster of fine wines may spend years developing them. Many of these people sense more than the mundane world through their ability; they also sense psychically through the mechanism of taste.

Clairolfaction: Here the person senses mainly by smell. They are able to distinguish by smell one individual from all others; they can also sense the smell of love, the smell of fear, and so on. Dogs of course have this sense developed to a very high degree. Women seem to have it more than men do.

Clairsentience: These people simply "feel" things in an emotional way. They are hard put to explain why a certain room or a certain place does not feel right. They don't see pictures or hear things to explain their hunches. Women often have this sense more developed than men do; this is why women are said to be emotionally reactive.

Everyone's abilities are slightly different. If we put numbers on them, one person may be 90 percent clairvoyant, 5 percent clairaudient, and 5 percent clairsentient. Another person may be only 10 percent clairvoyant and 10 percent clairaudient, but 80 percent clairsentient. This is why the same event affects people differently. The emotional impact of a piece of music may be very powerful to one person but felt hardly at all by another.

It is the aim of Tantra to develop all your senses so that you can fully comprehend any given object or event. The most mundane rock that you pick up in the garden emanates to all the senses. It is not just visible; it puts out sounds, it has a definite touch feeling, you can taste and smell it, you can feel its emotional background. When you are able to sense the rock with all the facets of your awareness, it will have far more beauty and significance to you than it had when it was just another rock; and the beauties of nature will be far more impressive when you use all your senses to become aware of them than when you viewed them passively.

It is also true that when you are fully aware and compose a Tantric ritual while in that state, you will be able to balance its sensory impact so that those who principally only hear or smell, for instance, will be as satisfied at the end of the ritual as those who see it.

It is your task as a neophyte Tantrist to develop all your senses and to extend the abilities of those senses that are already well developed. We therefore break the work into training for each of the six modes of awareness and into two subsections within each of the six. The first subsection covers methods to extend your awareness of the mundane (physical) world, and the second develops your awareness of the psychic world.

Think for a moment of the cave of a brown bear that has been hibernating all winter. The cave is now growing warm because spring has come, and the hibernating bear is waking up. What is your main impression of this event? Do you think of it as a picture of a bear in a cave? The rank smell of the bear? Do you hear him moving around? Do you feel the rough fur? Does a taste come into your mouth? Are you aware of his hunger pangs? Of course by thinking about it you can realize each of the senses; but what was your *first* reaction to the suggestion? Whatever mode you first thought about it in, that is your primary mode of awareness. In most people that mode is clairvoyance; but in many people one of the other senses is strongest.

YOUR AWARENESS TRAINING GUIDE

The following section will acquaint you with methods you can use to extend your sensory capability and improve your perception of the mundane objects around you. First you'll learn to train your mundane and then your psychic senses.

Visualization

Physical: Sit quietly in a comfortable chair when you have no
pressing tasks on your mind. Visualize as completely as you can
the growth and death of a lotus. Start inside the seed. See the
cell divisions going on. See the shoot break out of the seed
casing. See it push its way through the earth. See the tiny
seedling grow. Imagine it in all changing light and weather conditions. Finally see the flower come out. See the petals open.
Look into the beautiful interior of the lotus blossom. Now
watch as its petals fall and only the short stalk is left. Watch this
as it forms its seeds, then dies, completing the cycle. With practice you will become able to see this growth and death in every
minute detail.

Now visualize the face of your dyadic partner: every curve,
every blemish, every beauty spot, every expression. Sketch it
from memory.

Now think of walking around the house. See every detail of
every room. Get your partner to blindfold you, and walk
around the house using only your visualization ability to guide
you.

These exercises should be done once a day for a week, then
at least once a week, as you continually improve your visualization skills.

Psychic: You probably dream in pictures, but when you wake
you completely forget what pictures you saw. Many of the pictures have meaning to you, and come not from within your own
consciousness but from outside sources of awareness. Therefore
you should first learn to record dream pictures; then learn to
record the pictures you get in meditation. To start with, all you
need to do is keep a notebook handy and write down a few
simple notes on what you saw. As your skills grow, the notes
should be extended and sketches added of the things you saw.

Tantrists have a very simple way of developing the range of
eye vision. Often when you meet them they will seem to be
looking beyond you because they are using the Tantric method

of defocusing the vision to look at your psychic emanations. The same defocusing of the vision can be used to see emanations from any object. To start with, take these three steps:

1) Get a dyadic couple who are in the middle of the sexual fast to help you.

2) In a room where the light level is reduced, or against a dark background, have the two of them stand facing each other about two feet apart with fingertips almost touching.

3) Sit quietly three or four feet away. Close one eye. With the other eye look at the background BEHIND the nearly-touching fingertips. After a time you will begin to see a light purplish or white disturbance in the normal coloration of the background, caused by the flow of energy from one fingertip to the other. It may resemble a heating of the air between the fingertips. If you don't see anything with that eye, close it and look with the other eye. You will find that one eye gives better results than the other; however, once you recognize the effect, you will be able to look with both eyes and still see it.

The secret of this is not to look at the physical object but to look beyond it. Once you can readily detect the energy between the fingertips, you will be able to detect energies in differing circumstances. If you continue with the same dyadic couple, you will find that as the month goes by, so the color and the intensity of the energy between the fingertips vary. You will become able to tell, for instance, whether they are getting along well together in their work or having difficulty.

The Aura

For centuries it has been known that objects are surrounded by a field of energy, perceptible to many people as light. This is especially true of living objects, with animals (including humankind) displaying the most marked fields. In earlier times such

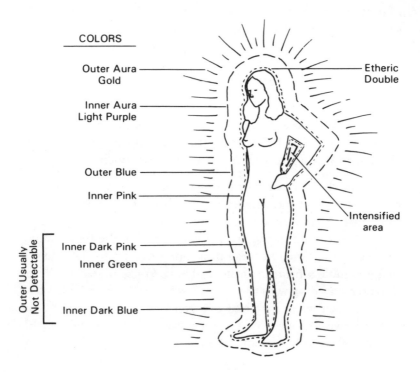

Figure 12.   The aura.

fields were called the "human atmosphere" or the "atmosphere of life"; the term aura is now generally used to describe them.

The first giant step forward in seeing auras was made in the mid-1800s, when it was discovered that by looking through a screen painted with dicyanin, anyone could see the aura. The recent discovery of Professor Kirlian—that it is possible to photograph the human aura when it interacts with an electrical field—has given new impetus to the study of the aura and to the use of Kirlian photographs, as they are called, to aid in diagnosis of illnesses of the body and of the mind. To see actual auras is simple. We suggest you proceed as follows:

1) Arrange a room so that it can be fully darkened, with one window where the light level can be easily adjusted to give varying low levels of diffused light. (Adjusting a blind behind a curtain is an easy way to arrange this.)

2) Get a friend[1] to stand against a matte black background (perhaps a dyed sheet) so that as you stand with your back to the window you can see him or her dimly.

3) If possible, ask your subject to strip to the waist. Then ask him or her to put hands on hips.

4) Look carefully with your better eye (as determined earlier) at the area between his or her rib cage and arm. Gradually dim the light until the subject is not visible but the field or aura is. Five minutes for this test is a long time, because the eyes tend to become tired.

5) Once you have seen the aura between the subject's arm and rib cage, look at the shoulder close to the head. You should be able to see another aura in this area.

6) After a week's experimenting of this sort, you should be able to see the total aura of people in almost any light.

Figure 12 shows what you can expect to see when you view the aura. Starting closest to the body, a very narrow dark transparent space extends maybe a quarter- to a half-inch from the body. Because it is so close to the body, this "etheric double" is often obscured by bulky clothing. Next you will see the inner aura, which, though transparent, is the densest part; then, fading away, the outer aura. This is quite variable in size, sometimes extending no more than an inch or two, and sometimes extend-

---

[1]Some sources recommend you view a child; but we suggest you work with a young adult as your subject because often a child's aura is wildly variable and difficult to see.

ing many feet. You may also see dark patches in the aura, rays of light extending across it, and even flecks of light in it.

The aura may be composed of various colors. As usual, the meaning of the colors will depend on what various colors mean to you in your reality. Table 3 shows the normal color gradation of a healthy aura as perceived by most people. The golden halo, of course, is the thing that medieval painters depicted in pictures of saints. This can be so strong that it becomes visible to almost everyone. For example, when an initiation "takes," the aura is bright for several days after the event. This caused one of our students much embarrassment during homeward travel after her initiation. She could see everyone was staring at her, so she went to the ladies' room and asked the attendant whether there was something wrong with her clothing. Being reassured on this score, she was finally set at ease by a stewardess who asked her, "Who are you? You have a golden halo. What is it? Are you a saint?"

Certain other characteristics of the aura can give important clues. Where you see black areas you should suspect there are

Table 3. Traditional Colors in the Aura

Color	Meaning
Black (sometimes with red flashes)	Hate
Lurid red	Sensuality
Crimson	Love
Orange-red	Pride
Yellow	Intellect, mental activity
Reddish-brown	Selfish lust
Brown	Avarice
Dirty blue	Selfishness
Deep blue-green	Sympathy
Gray-green	Cunning, deceit
Brownish green	Jealousy
Leaden gray	Depression
Light blue-gray	Fear

diseased parts. Black areas behind the ears mean drug problems. An open cone of light shaped as if it were made from wire indicates great fear.

Aura seeing is fun. It can be most helpful in your daily life since it enables you to gauge the mood of someone you are with and adjust your approach accordingly. It is also fun to use the ability in your normal workaday life, but be careful that people do not become too aware of your defocused look. They might suspect you are drunk or "stoned."

Hearing

Physical: In a manner similar to the way you watched a seed develop into a lotus, imagine yourself sitting by a small stream in a forest glen on a warm afternoon when there is a lot of insect activity. Imagine each sound in turn: the buzz and whine of the insects, the rustle of the leaves, the rippling of the water, and eventually the sound the plants make as they grow and the sound of the fish swimming. When you have all this sound information clearly in your mind, get a friend to blindfold you and take you to a local park. Sit still in a glade for ten minutes or so. Then ask the friend to take you home. Now find the exact place you were sitting.

Psychic: Again you need someone to help you. Your partner will perform three distinct exercises.

1) Have your partner stand before you and slowly almost-clap, not quite letting the hands meet. As the hands come together, you should hear a distinct "buzzing" sound. When you are fairly certain that you can hear it, have your partner do it behind your back and try to recognize when his or her hands are together or apart.

2) Have your partner put hands out with one palm up and one palm down, then turn slowly on his or her axis. This should produce a very slow "waa waa" sound. The highest intensity will be when each palm in turn is open toward you. Again, have

your partner do this behind you so you can tell from your psychic senses when either hand is actually pointing at you.

3) Sit in a low chair and have your friend extend hands toward you with palms down as he or she alternately squats and rises. In this way the energy field crosses your head as the fingertips move up and down. Again you should hear a "waa waa," but it is of much higher intensity and its peaks coincide with the instant when the fingers are level with your head. Again, once you have identified the sound, have your partner do it behind you.

Tantric students report that once they have developed their psychic hearing ability, they are annoyed by such things as fluorescent lamps and the hum from power and telephone lines. This is why all major power lines should be turned off in the area of a ritual.

Olfaction

Physical: Start by identifying widely different smells. Get four small containers: one in which a clove has been crushed, one in which some sulphur has been burned, one in which some lavender has been crushed, and one in which some garlic has been crushed. You should be able to detect the differences among these four odors. The trick now is to detect the distinctions between more subtle odors. One pleasant way of doing this is to get two or three people of the opposite gender to line up before bathing, and being blindfolded, smell the nape of each neck. As you develop your sense, you should become able to distinguish each individual by scent.

Psychic: Development of this sense is not easy if you have no natural bent for it. Getting yourself into situations which cause "smells of fear" and "smells of anger" can be a challenge. Hence you will probably find you must be content with smelling emotions of less strength.

How can you cut out your other senses while you test that of olfaction? You need the help of a dyadic couple, and you must cover up your sense of hearing with music and your etheric sight by viewing a TV program with the sound turned off. Have the couple display various emotions to each other, first perhaps touching each other in a loving way, then coupling. As this progresses, you should smell the sweetness of the emotions up to the point of coupling, when there should be a sudden change in your awareness. This is difficult; it is a subtle sense, but once developed, it can be very useful, especially in your dealings with animals.

Taste

Physical: The easiest and best-known set of tastes available are various wines and spirits. When you taste a wine, write down what physical flavor it has to your palate. In other words, give yourself a code word for its taste. You might say it tastes musty, or tastes the way gas smells, or some other code which is meaningful to you. Of course you can say it tastes acid or sour or vinegary. Then after eating a small piece of plain unsalted cracker or bread, taste another wine and again write down in your own words what it tastes like. Very soon you will be able to identify three or four different wines; then you will extend the capability to perhaps a dozen. At this point you can have a lot of fun with your friends. Some smart-alec wine connoisseurs (wine snobs) you will find cannot taste the difference between a red and a white! Beer drinkers who swear that only "this" brand is for them, when given three or four cold glasses of different beers are absolutely unable to identify them.

With spirits, the situation is even more remarkable. After the first taste of the first spirit, the taste buds are dulled by the alcohol and cannot detect wide differences in flavor. If you are ever challenged to identify various spirits, dilute each one with a large amount of water. Then you will have a reasonable chance of detecting the differences.

Psychic: A method widely used for testing taste is the enclosing of various objects in plastic and placing them in the mouth. You can try such things as a finger-ring that forms a closed circle; a finger-ring with a break in it; a piece of red paper; a piece of white. Each object has a different "taste." Gradually you will learn to distinguish among them.

Touch

Physical: To develop your physical sense of touch, all you need is the description of what something you touch REALLY feels like. Touch a piece of sandpaper and write down what it really feels like. No, you can't get away with saying just "rough." You need to write at least a sentence. Now touch a piece of glass. Write what it will feel like to touch the surface of some very cold water; then go and do it. You may be surprised that it doesn't really feel like that. Next write what a piece of silk or some other texture feels like to touch, and see whether your Tantric co-workers can identify the object you are describing. Eventually you will know what something will feel like before you touch it, and when blindfolded can make your way around the group and identify various members by touching their foreheads or their hair.

Psychic: Probably the most famous psychic of modern times is Peter Hurkos. He uses tactition—psychometry—in his work. Every object has its own psychic feel. Take a tablecloth from a

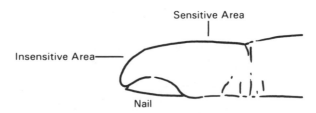

Figure 13. Areas of sensitivity on the finger.

gourmet meal and cut it into two pieces. Wash one half very carefully and have a dyadic couple put it between them during ritual copulation. By lightly touching the two pieces of fabric, then, you should be able easily to distinguish their different emanations.

It is also true that every color has its own emanation. If you hold a brightly printed plastic-wrapped package, as you move your fingertip across the surface you will grow able to detect when you move from one color to another.

From a glossy magazine select pictures that display strong clear patches of various colors. From the pictures cut pieces of four different colors. Put them into a linen bag which is big enough to receive your entire hand. Now down in the linen bag, without looking at them, feel each piece of paper in turn between your thumb and fingertip and see whether you can sense which color is which. It may take you several sessions to get the right color each time; but this practice will pay off handsomely in your future psychometric work, so persist until your accuracy is high.

These tips will help you learn to read colors:

1) Figure 13 shows the area of your fingertip most sensitive for psychometric work. Notice that it is not the tip of the finger but the lower portion of the pad. This is the area you should use to touch the pieces of colored paper in your practice sessions.

2) Your various fingers have differing degrees of sensitivity. Normally the most sensitive is your longest finger; but if your fingers are of about the same length, they probably all have about the same level of sensitivity.

3) Power flows out of your hands, especially out of the palms. You have already learned how to impress your emotions on an object. Now, though, it's important to avoid imprinting the object you want to read with fresh, irrelevant emotions of your own. For instance, if you pick up a piece of colored paper in

your linen-bag practice and think very strongly, "This one is the red piece," you may impress on that piece of paper red emanations to such an extent that it will feel red to you from then on. This impressed-emanation problem is much diminished if you use your secondary hand[2] in psychometric work. To avoid confusion, replace your practice scraps of paper after every four or five sessions.

4) You are more sensitive to receiving information through your fingers when you are in a homeostatic condition. To gain this condition you should a) adjust the room temperature to a level at which you are comfortable; b) work after a light meal rather than after a heavy one; c) be emotionally at peace—there is no point in trying this test if you are being pushed into it by someone else or if you are angry or sexually uptight, because any of these things will tend to disguise the results you should be getting from your fingertips; d) arrange your body to be unbound—if, for instance, you have on your wrist a bracelet heavily laden with past emotions, the very weak emanations from the papers of various colors will never get past your wrist to your head. Instead they will be wholly absorbed in the emotional output of the bracelet. The same is true of such things as wedding rings, or in fact any binding on the body. Women should be especially aware that metal hair-fasteners can totally disrupt their efforts at psychometry, and should remove all such objects.

It takes only a few moments to arrange yourself so that you can try the color-detector test. Once you have learned how to detect the four different colored paper scraps, you will use the same technique to do such things as psychometrize the name of the stock that will gain the most for you in the market, or which companion will be the most enjoyable on a date. Practice and learn. Learn how easy it really is.

---

[2]See chapter 2.

Sentition

Physical: Sentition experiments are difficult because the area around you must be "clean" and you yourself must be very relaxed. If you have a natural ability for sentition, try to help the other members of the group by describing as best you can what you "feel" in certain situations. If you don't have the ability and have no one really to help you, sit down and write out what you feel—not when you are angry (for example), but when there is anger near you. In a similar way, write out what you feel when there is love near you; and as the third point of the triangle, write out what you feel when there is hate near you.

Psychic: Again it is best to have a dyadic couple help you. You must cover up your other sensory inputs as you did in working toward developing your clairolfaction. Music, TV pictures, incense, and placing your hands in cool water are all considered essential training aids.

Have the dyadic couple stand behind you, and let them face each other while each holds one hand of the other. Ask them to put their free hands one on each side of your head but not touching it. Now have a third person show them each in turn a picture of a flower, a picture of a couple making love, and a picture of a lion eating its prey. It is up to you to detect which picture they are looking at.

Developing and strengthening your psychometric ability needs practice; the first exercise to that end will serve as a foundation for nearly all your psychometric work. It is your basic fingertip detector.

We have found no better test of this etheric sentition ability than this one. From your local five-and-dime, buy twelve identical pearl shirt buttons. Obtain a piece of black fabric about a foot square, the same size fabric in white silk, a paperback book on Satanism or some other very negative subject, a book of light-hearted cartoons (perhaps a Peanuts book or a Garfield), and a package of plain white envelopes. Put six of the buttons into an envelope and into the negative book, and wrap the book in the black fabric. Put the other six buttons into the light-hearted book and wrap it in the white fabric. In the Western world, of course, black is "evil" and white is "good;" and what you are trying to do is impress negative and positive emanations on the sets of buttons.

Let each package remain undisturbed for a week or so before you try your sentition ability on them. Now hold each button in turn in your secondary hand. See whether you can detect which ones are good and which are evil. This effort may be enhanced if you hold the button at the center of your forehead, using the palm of your secondary hand to do so. Continue this experiment until you can detect the differences in the buttons.

THE COLOR OF YOUR OUTPUT

You should be careful in selecting clothing. Think about the clothes you are wearing at this moment. Does each garment have good feelings, or are some of them so-so, and some perhaps actually negative? This has little to do with the physical colors of the garments, although the colors will affect other people and may key your own head to a particular response when you see your reflection in a mirror. If you are wearing a light yellow sweater, that sweater will tend to put out emanations of light-hearted "sunny" feelings. But if you wore that same sweater when something very negative happened to you, the sweater may be putting out not only its natural light-hearted emanations; it may be emitting emanations from the negative event as well. The sweater might also bear negative feelings imprinted into it before you ever bought it. Maybe it was a factory second, or the seamstress who made it was in a vile mood as it lay in her hands. Any of these things will tend to color the sweater psychically so that it influences you and the people you meet.

Maybe you are wearing a sexy pair of jeans that ought to be putting out good green sexual emanations to attract the opposite gender; but what if you broke up with your former lover in a very emotional scene on that last date—in these jeans—or had to reject the advances of some unattractive and aggressive slob? Then the psychic color of the jeans will not be what you might wish. In such a case, though you may have a perfect color combination on the physical plane, the psychic emanations may be horrible; thus everyone you meet would be turned off by your clothing, even though they might not know why they feel that way.

Try laying out your clothing on the bed and reading each garment psychometrically for good and bad feelings, using the sensitivity you developed when you psychometrically analyzed your shirt-button-envelope combinations. You will want to identify and wear only those clothes that will make you look good; that is, the clothes that give you good psychic "color." Usually there is no need actually to discard clothing with negative emanations. Peter Hurkos and other noted psychics report that if you send a negative-radiating garment to the cleaners twice in a row, the emanations are removed from it and are no longer at such a level of intensity that they affect you or your acquaintances.

Until you can get your clothes shaped up or replaced (no amount of cleaning will remove the emanations from a garment made of badly woven fabric), wear only those clothes that feel good. Your world will suddenly become brighter as people feel more friendly toward you.

PART
TWO

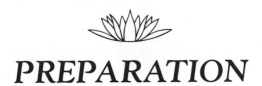

PREPARATION

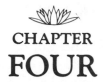

CHAPTER
FOUR

Meditating on the Lotus

THE LOTUS IS the Eastern symbol of duality and transcendence. The thrusting spike develops into the beautiful opening flower with its central thrusting stamen. The symbolic lingam and yoni that the lotus represents produce great beauty. Each petal is part of your spiritual understanding, yet the stem anchors it to the earth. In this mode the lotus represents the growth of understanding from humble soil and water. If made fertile with muck, the muck makes the growth of the lotus more healthy and vigorous, ascending from its filthy beginnings to achieve beauty.

The force comes from within you, from your mundane body, the "Me." By its use you can achieve many marvelous things such as healing. Yet in healing or using the force to help you through your life, you are developing your spirit, the real you, the "I." So the lotus also represents the duality of "I" and "Me" in one.

"I" AND "ME"—THE DUALITY WITHIN YOU

Almost from your first breath you have lived with the duality of the spirit living in the body-shell: "I" and "Me." In some ways there is conflict between the two parts of your being; yet each needs the other. "Me" is the source of physical demands. It is constantly pushing at you, demanding attention. "Me" wants to be fed. "Me" wants to get laid. "Me" wants the pretty trinket in the store.

In contrast "I" has no need of such things—but "I" knows that without "Me" "I" would have nowhere on this plane of existence to dwell. Therefore it behooves "I" to give in occasionally to "Me." "Me" also knows that without "I" it is nothing, so it resists the separation of "I" from "Me."

One of the main purposes of Tantra is to teach you to separate "I" from "Me" and to develop each separately. Spiritual strengthening comes from releasing the spirit during satiation. Strengthening of the will and "Me" comes through controlled abstinence. Two different types of meditation are used for this type of development training.

Meditation of the first type is sometimes called single-pointed or lotus-stem. It is designed to raise your force and to teach you to control body functions. This is the type of meditation made popular by the proponents of Transcendental Meditation and other such systems. Martial artists learn it. Its whole idea is to focus all the attention into a single point for one instant in time. This meditation seeks to give the person supernormal abilities for an instant (not supernatural abilities, just supernormal). There are countless stories of people who have lifted cars off small children and endured pain of all kinds by using this single-pointed type of meditation. Through it you can develop your force to new highs.

The other type, which we are finally becoming aware of in the West, is called lotus-petal meditation. As the lotus petals open, they reach upward and outward, gathering in the sunlight and the dewy moisture that give them life. You, too, can reach outward and develop spiritual communication and gain psychic energy which will revitalize your life.

To be successful in petal meditation, you have to convince "Me" to stop wanting mundane things; for so long as "Me" is clamoring to have its demands met "I" can never communicate with IT or with other spirits. In some ways this is like a parent trying to get away on a private errand—one that an obstreperous child is trying to prevent. Every time the parent wants time to him- or herself, the child screams bloody murder, falls down frothing at the mouth, or even breaks a bone to prevent the parent's departure.

"Me" is a very tough customer. It's been looking out for itself against the world for the whole of your life. "Me" has the firm opinion that if "I" turns its back, "Me" will become possessed or maybe die; and "Me" doesn't want to die. It has all those good bodily appetites still to fulfill. What you have to do, therefore, is convince "Me" that "I" having its own time represents no threat and will actually be beneficial to "Me" because during "I's" trip it will be looking for things that will help "Me" satisfy its appetites. What you eventually end up doing is making a bargain between the two halves of yourself.

When you want to go single-pointed, you suppress "I" and let "Me" have free rein. When you want to be spiritual, you satisfy the majority of "Me's" immediate demands and then say, "Now it's time for 'I'. If you don't let 'I' go, 'I' will be mad at 'Me' and in future will not satisfy 'Me's' appetites."

Another metaphor for the two types of meditation is that of a man with a garden. Imagine his small garden, beautifully nurtured and tended. He surrounds it with a moat. Inside the moat he builds a strong wall. Within the confines of the wall he finds strength. He loves his garden and tends it with great care. Gradually he comes to concentrate on the perfection of the well at the center of the garden.

Eventually he metaphorically goes inside the well, concentrating his whole being inside it. He even goes down into the water of the well, into the dark places of his own consciousness, and in the bottom of the well he finds a pinpoint of bright light caused by the sunlight striking down through the water. He concentrates his entire consciousness on that one bright light. When everything, every particle of his being is focused on that one point, he is doing single-pointed meditation.

At other times he looks outward from his garden. He finds the world is a noisy smelly place containing people and things that he cannot control. It worries him and he draws back. But eventually he looks again. He sees that many of the things and beings which he cannot control are just like himself, that many of the fears he had are within his own mind. Gradually he learns to accept them. All the monsters, all the gargoyles, all the things that go bump in the night, all are accepted as part of the world outside the garden wall. Slowly and tentatively he reaches further outward, further into the unknown. He breaks down the wall that encircles his understanding. Hesitantly, then with more confidence, he reaches upward and outward and learns of everything contained in the space outside his garden.

The metaphor of the garden shows the clear difference between lotus-stem and lotus-petal meditation. Many say that when you reach outward far enough you come to a point of light and that through the wormholes of the space/time continuum this point of light is connected to the point of light at the bottom of the well. All is one. One is all.

LOTUS-STEM MEDITATION

To understand perfect concentration, think of the six aspects or six modes through which every creature and every object expresses itself:

1) It is visible;

2) It makes a sound;

3) It has a smell;

4) It has a taste or flavor;

5) It has a texture;

6) It has its own psyche (is alive) or has impressed on it a psychic feeling.

When you fully experience an object or a living creature, you use all these six modes of understanding. In full meditation of an object, you first visualize, then hear, then taste, then feel, then smell, and then sense the feeling of the whole object. In some people only one or two of these sensory inputs are developed. As a student of Tantra, your goal will be to develop all inputs until you can become one with the object being sensed. In doing a ritual, you *become* the object of the ritual: the healing pulse, the money on its way to you, the lover, whatever.

Let's try a practical experiment. Perhaps you have in your fruit bowl a pear or an apple you would enjoy. Let's see whether you can improve its flavor and texture. Hold the fruit in your hands. Smell its ripeness. Feel the warmth of the sun it has absorbed. Taste in your mouth the most perfect luscious pear or apple you've ever eaten, and project this taste into the fruit. Listen to the song of the fruit tree in your mind. Experience the aliveness of the fruit. Think of the seed within that you will plant when you have eaten the fruit.

Now slowly take the first bite. It is indeed the best bite of fruit you've ever had. Through concentration you have made the fruit perfect, exactly as you want it to be. Continue to eat and enjoy your fruit. You worked at it; you deserve the pleasure. If you think this way of eating fruit does not enhance your enjoyment, simply eat a piece absentmindedly and then eat one while you meditate on it.

Sealing-in-Stem Meditation

The sealing-in-stem meditation is used to retain the developed energy within the body until it bursts forth at the direction of your will. With the fingers of both hands, touch in this order your forehead, your eyes, nose, mouth, ears, solar plexus. With each touch imagine the lotus closing back into its spear. If you like, you may think with each touch, "I am sealed and protected." This is a sealing to keep energy in. If you like, you can imagine yourself sealed in a tight sphere of light. Now place the hands, palms down, on the thighs or put them together in the traditional prayer attitude.

Lotus-Stem Meditation, Male Practice

This single-pointed meditation exercise is designed to focus and concentrate the whole being. The exercise uses the genitalia as the focusing point. Sitting with his back perfectly vertical[1] and with his dyadic partner close by, the yogi directs his detailed concentration to the yoni, visualizing it in all six of its aspects. It is pictured usually with lovely flower-like labia, the clitoris vibrant and healthy, erect, and the vagina itself gently opening and closing like a flower, inviting the entry of the lingam. Clearly if a lingam touches this opening and closing yoni it will be sucked in gently but firmly.

The texture of the yoni is next experienced, soft and warm, moist and welcoming. Then he concentrates on the scent of the feminine essence. Understanding the sensation of smell of the female is very important in this meditation. During the sacred rites, a little musk is often placed on the yoni; it is this musky odor that must be called to mind. The yoni has its own fresh, soft flavor, the essence of the female. Once experienced by the male, it is never forgotten. This soft musk taste is one of the most powerful mind stimulants that a male can use, provided it has been experienced in conjunction with positive and happy sexual times. The sound of the yoni is next experienced. Many find this difficult to achieve at first. It is the sound of the heartbeat, the hollow, deep drum rhythm that can occasionally be heard when a large bass drum is very gently tapped. It is a slow rhythm, an earth rhythm, that pulses with life.

---

[1]You may need to sit against a wall or a tree. Few Westerners can achieve the Eastern sitting position and maintain it with sufficient comfort to meditate.

Lastly the whole feeling of the yoni is experienced: the mother, the lover, and the nymph feeling combined into one. It is both pleasure and pain. In meditation it is natural for the male to concentrate on the pleasure aspect. As more meditation is done and skills are strengthened, the level of awareness expands and the pleasure aspect is replaced with total understanding. Through that understanding the male perfects his yonic caresses.

When the single-pointed meditation is done correctly, within less than a minute the male will be totally erect and hard. Many males can ejaculate purely with this meditation, or at most with a touch of the fingertip from the female partner gently and softly caressing the very underside tip of the lingam. The intent of the meditation is to get to the point of climax and stay there without actually climaxing for 32 minutes.

Lotus-Stem Meditation, Female Practice

The female also uses single-pointed meditation, focusing on the lingam. First it is visualized, as erect, ready, with the foreskin drawn back so that the coral head with its typical mushroom shape is visible. She thinks carefully of each detail in turn, examining the hard, vibrant condition, the smooth baby-skin texture of the tip, the rougher texture of the stem. The texture is experienced as though it were touching the clitoris or the clitoris were exploring it. In the interior eye the feeling of the clitoris rubbing against the stem is experienced; in fact the stem is not felt with the finger but only with the clitoris.

She brings to mind the flavor of the tiniest drop of seminal fluid. The sense of taste is a very powerful one; in some females the flavor of seminal fluid is a turn-off, but Tantrists learn to make it a turn-on. Only in Western culture is seminal fluid regarded as something vaguely unpleasant. It is in fact a power-

ful antibiotic containing no bacteria or other harmful organ-
isms, so it is beneficial to bring the taste to mind and retain it.

Now the male smell is brought to mind. In India, patchouli
incense is used on the lingam before the sacred coupling. If you
cannot bring the essence of the male to mind, imagine patchouli
instead. The fact that this scent is indelibly imprinted on your
consciousness in association with pleasurable sexual activity will
intensify the effectiveness of the meditation.

Experience now the sound of the lingam. Its throbbing beat
is faster than the deep earth tones of the Mother. It is insistent;
it is sharp. It will not go away until it slowly melds with your
own female slower earth tones.

Now experience the vibrant thrusting nature of the lingam.
If you like, imagine it inside you: its thrusting vibrancy, the male
sword of pleasure, the essence of the male creative aspect. The
feeling is one of the sun's heat and life.

As with the male, female one-pointed meditation can bring
the experienced yogin right to the point of orgasm. It is said in
the old scriptures that at this point a single touch of the lingam
would push her over the edge into orgasm. She, too, tries to
maintain this state for 32 minutes.

Practice both these single-pointed meditations for longer
and longer periods of time so that a single touch or the insertion
of the lingam into the yoni immediately brings about orgasm. It
is a vitally important skill in Tantric Yoga.

Notice that in this exercise the male thinks of the yoni in his
own terms—and the female of the lingam in her own terms.
Through this meditative understanding each becomes an infinitely better lover.

MASTURBATION AND MEDITATION

As society's list of taboos grows shorter, so increasing numbers
of Tantrists use a form of masturbation to help their lotus-stem
meditation along, bringing themselves physically to the point of

orgasm before going into meditation. This approach may be excellent for novices, but serious practitioners believe it detracts from the training of "Me." Tantric work is best done with a partner; the loving feelings and bondings that are established between partners working in this way are irreplaceable.

IDA AND PINGALA

When you have learned the basic stem meditation, deliberately slow down your breathing as you maintain yourself on the edge of climax. With one of your senses you will feel power being generated in the genitalia and flowing up the spine into the head. Your head may feel hot or overfilled or "aching" or just ready. The most common sensation is that of seeing or feeling a red and a gold intertwined spiral of light ascending from your genitalia, joining together, and merging in your head. These streams are the Male and Female Principles—the Ida and Pingala. If you are a male and stem-meditate on the female, the Female Principle enters your consciousness and both ascend. If you are a female and stem-meditate on the Male Principle, it comes to you and both ascend. Each needs the other to gain release. Until you welcome the opposite principle and understand it, nothing will work.

Those who regularly practice this stem meditation open up their consciousness to the forces of the opposite gender. The male gains more understanding of the female and the female more understanding of the male. When this type of meditation has been carried on for a long time, it can be expanded to include more characteristics of the other gender. Gradually the male opens fully to the Female Principle and the female opens fully to the Male Principle. Thus consciousness within each is expanded, and instead of being at two opposite poles they become one.

As the meditations progress, the presence of the God and Goddess Principles will grow stronger. You may start to tremble or have light muscle spasms like mini-climaxes. When this stage manifests, you must send the force to do your bidding. Clap your hands, yell, shout, command the force to go and do what you want. It should burst through the top of your head in a ball of blue-white light. At the same time or within a fraction of a second, a climax should occur; then you can expect to blank out completely and lose consciousness. You will awake tired but somehow refreshed, sexually exhausted but ready for more. This is yet another duality of feelings, but one which brings with it a fantastic time of learning for "Me," for new knowledge will come to you from your own unconscious.

MAITHUNA TRAINING

During the Tantric ritual of Maithuna, the lingam is within the yoni but ejaculation is forbidden. In the usual first position the female lies on her back; her legs are intertwined with the male's, and he enters her very deeply and solidly while lying on his side. When the partners are trained, any and all sexual positions are used. In Maithuna, it is taboo to use the hands to arouse the partner, though partners are allowed to grasp and stroke each other's forearms and to suck their fingers. The genitalia should move slowly, the yoni milking and the lingam thrusting and rhythmically expanding. Each tries to get the other to climax; it is a very adult game. This is the pleasure-pain Tantric training system of control. It is not really a meditation.

The Tantrist can learn to have an orgasm through meditation alone, and can also learn not to have an orgasm no matter what is happening to the genitalia. It is said that all sensations are experienced only in the mind, and that the pleasurable sensations associated with sex are the same as those associated with pain. If you can control the sexual sensation, you can control the pain sensation.

In the Maithunic ritual, control is maintained for 32 minutes. Describing this mind exercise is extremely difficult. The paradox in Maithunic meditation is that the turn-on must be maintained while not thinking about it. Many workers simply concentrate on a single-pointed white light; others draw a very complex mandala or diagram and concentrate on each aspect of it. The guru recommends concentrating on a white light or on the intertwined red and gold spirals near the spine. You start to concentrate on the white light when you are near orgasm, enjoying all the pleasurable sensations, all the things that are happening to you. Only when you come close to orgasm do you use your will to withdraw from it, trying to become one with the partner and one with the light. The male has the more challenging task. It is advised in the writings that if he is very close he should stop breathing. This stoppage of breath prevents the semen flowing. The breath is not stopped by closing the throat but by holding the throat open. At first, for a few moments when the breath is stopped and the pleasurable sensations continue, it seems as if nothing can prevent orgasm; but gradually as it becomes more and more difficult to keep the breath stopped, and as he feels every aspect of the white light blazing inside his head, the orgasmic impulse recedes and calmness and oneness are brought to the act.

When they first practice the sacred rite, many couples remain totally still. But as they get further along the path they begin to play games with each other, trying to make the other have an orgasm while refraining themselves. Some couples can hold close to orgasmic peak for much longer than the 32-minute cycle, but all practitioners agree this is not the path. When the cycle is complete, the sacred books require pause while the mundane parts of the ritual are completed before either partner completes the orgiastic act. The guru strongly recommends that within a couple of hours after Maithuna a normal orgasm occur for both partners.

DAYDREAMING

In the rush of today's life, you rarely spend long times working at pursuits that allow your mind to drift free while the tasks keep the body occupied. When Grandpa followed the mule and plowed the field, he could meditate upon his life and think about other farm tasks. While Grandma's hands were busy washing the clothes, she, too, could become contemplative. One of today's most famous psychic teachers working in South America assigns people to carry heavy stones endlessly up hills. This great guru's modern discovery of an "aid to awareness" is just the rediscovery of ancient knowledge. The hands and body are kept busy with a task which requires no conscious attending; consequently the mind drifts free and the subconscious is able to bring through to the conscious mind the information it has been absorbing throughout the worker's lifetime. Since the tractor took over from the mule and the washing machine from the scrub board, people have continually packed more labor-saving devices into their homes; thus tasks which formerly allowed natural meditation have been eliminated.

One of the few tasks remaining is long-distance driving; another is weeding the garden. You should use these opportunities to relax, daydream if you will, and meditate, paying attention to all the information your subconscious mind is giving you. In many ways you owe yourself at least a half-hour a day to drift. Take the time to become serene. Let "I" and "Me" communicate. You deserve it!

LOTUS-PETAL MEDITATION

We have trained thousands in this method of meditation. It may not be the easiest system available, but we are altogether confident that our method is both effective and safe. So as you embark on this new experience, do not skip steps; follow the instructions exactly as they are given.

A Tantrist very rarely waits passively for anything, especially for direction along life's path. Vaguely hoping for a dream or a sign just isn't a very satisfactory way to run your life. During meditation, in addition to getting the two halves of your own self in contact with each other, you can also reach outward and upward to receive guidance on problems to which you do not know the answers. A great deal of information can also be gained from the spirits. You will most probably have one special spirit assigned to aid you in your work — your Guide. Because of the Law of Attraction, this will be someone whose ideas and tastes closely resemble yours.

If you plan never to work at more than the theory of Tantra, you do not absolutely have to meditate; but everyone, even the most hurried and harassed housewife, should set aside fifteen to thirty minutes every day for her own private time in which all pressures are off her, a time when she can relax.

In dreaming and in meditation, as your awareness increases, you will become aware of other dimensions of information available to you. This can be helpful in the mundane "paycheck" world, and you can reach out into the future to help yourself as well. You might think of it as plugging into the great Cosmic Consciousness to receive information that will make your future secure and serene.

PROTECTION

Because you are trying to open yourself just like a lotus blossom in order to receive all that golden knowledge out there, you must protect yourself against the unwanted intrusion of negative energies and spirits. First, of course, never open yourself when you are down or depressed or in any way sick or off-color.

You will only draw to yourself more of the negativity that is temporarily in you. "Me" is also very concerned about the safety of "I" (especially in the early months) and will try all sorts of tricks to prevent proper meditation unless appropriate protective measures are taken. This concern is overcome by "Me's" acknowledgment that you—that is, "I"—have already been open at night in dreams or "away" in astral travel.

"Me" has become increasingly concerned in recent years about the supposed horrors of possession. Movies, books, and whispered stories in the occult community all have made possession a lurid and very present threat to "Me." Protection of the psychic kind is the answer to this anxiety. Such protection must be on a level that "Me" understands; that is, it must be in the physical reality and it must convince other spirits that the meditator is protected.

Once you have contacted your Guide, protection becomes a secondary concern and the measures can be dropped. In these early months, though, *do not outwardly meditate without psychic protection.*

This is a very real warning. Though the technique of psychic protection is quite simple, it may seem a nuisance. People get into meditation and think they are above these simple procedures; but we have been involved in psychic research for a long time, and we tell you that every step of the protection is necessary. We still are scrupulous about doing protections, even after many years of training.

FIRST STEPS IN OUTWARD MEDITATION

If you were set the task of baking a cake but you had no equipment, not even a stove, and no kitchen to work in, you would need a considerable amount of time to assemble all the equipment necessary and get set up. The same is true of meditation.

Step 1

The first thing you need to do is to get yourself comfortable.

• Find a comfortable chair.[2] In it there must be no iron or steel or material of animal origin, and the very minimum of non-ferrous metal. Metals, especially ferrous metals, become magnetized. You are working with minute electrical and magnetic impulses, and all outside interference must be reduced to a minimum. Make sure the chair supports you so you can sit comfortably for fifteen minutes without moving. Sit in your chair and read a book, but don't move your body, only your hands and head. Are you really comfortable? If not, refine your arrangements until you are.

• Find a quiet-running mechanical timer. Nowadays most kitchens have such a timer. Check yours for running noise, because too loud a ticking has a hypnotic effect on some people.

• Find a loose flowing robe, pure white, made preferably from cotton or linen. Synthetic fabrics are not acceptable. A wraparound front-opening dressing gown is ideal. In climates where nudity is comfortable, this is preferable; but if cold distracts your mind, wear the robe.

• Find a container of salt.

Step 2

Select a place. Somewhere in your home there is a spot suitable for meditation. In order of importance the requirements are:

• a wall running approximately North/South;

• an area along this wall that is not near heavy electric cabling or appliances;

---

[2]If you can sit in lotus posture with no chair, this is also quite acceptable.

• an absolute minimum of clutter. Books and newspapers are especially undesirable because of the busy thought patterns they engender;

• a location as close to the sky as possible (outdoorish in feeling). In the South this might be a patio; in colder climates it might be the master bedroom.

Step 3

Establish a time and stick with it. The factors influencing your choice of time vary from individual to individual, but here are some things that should be considered.

• When can you be uninterrupted?

• Can you keep this appointment every day unless something unforeseen interferes?

• Will your mind be free of petty work and household problems during the chosen time? That is, is it far enough removed from outside distractions so you can let your mind float without being tugged back?

• The time you choose should be such that it is within one hour of sunrise or sunset.

Step 4

Now it's time for your trial run. Let us say you have selected dawn or 6 A.M. as your test period. Ideally you will have slept with a partner and are free of sexual tension. By morning most of life's cares have been dropped and are not so oppressive that they intrude. You are in the state we call homeostatic. For the trial run, get up about 5:45.

• Complete your purification and washing.[3]

---

[3]See chapter 5.

• Put on a clean robe and go to your selected area. Subdue the light.

• Use salt to draw an unbroken circle around you clockwise on the floor.

• Set the timer for five minutes. Sit facing either East or West. Have your legs uncrossed and your hands resting on your thighs with palms up; tilt your head very slightly back. Look up toward the ceiling. When you are settled and comfortable, absolutely relax all muscles in your body.

If there are annoyances such as noises or areas of bright light coming from sources beyond your control, you may have to change the time of meditation. Re-adjust the setting and set the timer for another five minutes. Try again. Your area and equipment may or may not be satisfactory now, because your sensitivity is increasing as your eyes would adjust to a darkened room. If you feel another spot in the home would be better, don't be afraid to change the location. You won't know until you try.

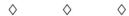

Continue these five-minute trials until you are satisfied that you have achieved the best conditions possible in your circumstances. This does not mean that you have to create a setting like a dark room at midnight. Your goal is relaxation and comfort—that's all.

Up to this point you have taken no protective measures, so ignore messages or impressions that arrive spontaneously. If a persistent thought occurs or a persistent picture is seen, immediately protect yourself as described in the next section, First Meditation, and start again. If the message is repeated, act on it. You are one of the lucky ones who receive immediately. This can happen when there is a buildup of information intended for you; the accumulated messages come through at the first opportunity. After a week or so, this initial burst will subside and you can start real work.

Now your preparations are complete, and you can proceed toward consistent communication. You are ready for your first genuine Tantra-style meditation.

FIRST MEDITATION

All your faculties are resting and waiting. You are in a state of homeostasis, with all your cravings moderately satisfied. There is nothing pulling or tugging at you, either mentally or physically.

Arrange the scene as you have experimentally determined it should be. With the salt shaker draw an unbroken circle of salt around you clockwise on the floor. If you are meditating in a carpeted area, spread a clean bedsheet first. The salt may be reused day after day, but you must cast the circle anew each time you meditate. Sit and make sure you are comfortably settled. Set the timer for fifteen minutes.

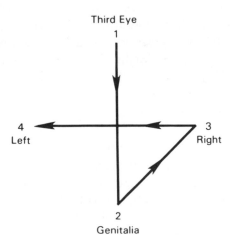

Figure 14.   Forming the equal-armed cross.

With eyes closed, say aloud:

> Spirits of mischievous intent,
> Spirits of lower entities,
> You cannot cross this sacred line.

Make the sign of the equal-armed cross by raising your right hand, and with your first and second fingers together touch your forehead (Third Eye). Sweep your hand straight down and touch your genitalia. Now move your hand up to chest level and to the right and touch your right shoulder; then sweep across the body from right to left and touch your left shoulder, as shown in figure 14. Say:

> May the Elder Ones protect me.
> I ask the protection of Shakti and Shiva.
> As they will, so let it be.

You now have around you a permanent protective forcefield resembling a white veil or halo of light. Mentally open this aura as you open your robe, laying aura and robe back simultaneously. Say:

> Guides, I am naked in your sight.
> My body and my mind are unclothed.
> Protect them, and send to me what you wish.

In order to encourage the spirits (many of whom were reared as Christians) and to protect yourself further, it is well to say a modified version of the Lord's Prayer. The modifications are minor, and the spirits feel comfortable in this environment.

> Our friends who are in Bliss:
> blessed be your names.
> God's dominion come.
> God's will be done on earth

as it is in Bliss.
Give us today our daily bread.
Forgive us our weaknesses
as we forgive those who wrong us.
Help us endure our trials,
and deliver us from negation.
So let it be.

Now begin the first mental exercise: the raising of a cone of power. Mentally picture a tall thin cone whose base rests in your lap and whose point disappears into the universe. The cone strengthens as it climbs your body. Concentrate on this concept a little while. You are putting out thought waves which resemble electromagnetic transmissions; they are capable of passing through any substance. The cone of power serves to conduct messages and impressions to you.

Open the lotus. Touch your forehead with the fingers of your right hand and the top of your head with the fingers of the left. Push your head slightly backward. Roll your eyes upward as if you are looking at the ceiling. Visualize the lotus opening as you lay back all your defenses and become totally open to the realms above. Without changing the position of head or eyes, rest your hands on your thighs, with palms upward and open, completely relaxed.

Now wait, expecting to receive messages, but not concentrating on anything. This is a difficult time for the beginner. Messages of many different types may be received. Most probably you will see messages visually—but you may also receive them through your sense of hearing, smell, touch, or taste. Think of a baseball park on a hot afternoon when someone has just hit a home run: Do you see, hear, smell, taste, or feel the scene? This same receptor sense usually (though not always) carries over into meditation.

It may happen at any time—a sudden flash of light or an inspiration. A common first sight is an eye watching you, through whose iris you can see new vistas. A common first feeling is to be drawn up out of the body, floating free where new things are felt and inspirations occur. Whatever happens, don't be startled. Let go. If a white flash occurs at the edge of your vision, indicating your Guide's presence, don't jerk your head around. The abrupt movement of your earth-plane shell will disturb reception, and you will break contact.

After a time that often seems too short, the bell of the timer sounds and you come back to the physical part of life. Common practice is the offering of a short healing prayer to use up the force built up within the cone of power and the salt ring. Say:

> I ask this great unseen healing force
> To remove all obstructions from my mind and body
> And to restore me to perfect health.
> I ask this in all sincerity and honesty,
> And I will do my part.

> I ask this great unseen healing force
> To bless both present and absent ones
> Who are in need of help,
> And to restore them to perfect health.
> I put my faith and trust in the love of the God.

During the first verse, imagine the cone of power dissolving into yourself and any companion(s). During the second verse, direct the remaining part of the cone to travel out to a specific person(s) in need.

Close your robe and your aura by imagining the closing of the lotus, while you affirm:

> I am surrounded by the pure white light of the God.
> Nothing but good shall come to me;
> Nothing but good shall go from me.
> I give thanks. So let it be.

Imagine the white veil once again enclosing you.

Follow Up

If you have a companion, talk now of what you each experienced. If you have no companion, write down any impression you received with the date of its occurrence. This will clear the message away to make room for new ones in your next sitting. If you find it difficult to come out of the meditative mood, at the close of the sitting drink a glass of water to which you have added a tablespoonful of vinegar and a tablespoonful of honey.

YOUR FLOW CHART OF OUTWARD MEDITATION

Figure 15 shows a step-by-step breakdown of this seemingly complex but actually simple procedure that we call outward meditation. It also includes a requirement to define your meditative goal. This can be as simple as wanting to communicate with a loved one, or as complex as wanting to know the true meaning of life.

Look at figure 15, starting at the top of the page at Step 1. This step is easy to accomplish. When you get to Step 2, however, you see there are two paths: either YES downward, leading toward Step 3, or NO. To the right of NO you see instructions to be followed to continue your development.

Following the steps in their logical sequence leads you naturally into your first contact with spirits. Be sure that you take these steps every time you meditate, even after you have established contact with your Guide.

GETTING IT WORKING

If nothing dramatic happens in their first few meditations, some people give up. We urge you to be persistent and notice how serene your life is becoming. Something dramatic will happen;

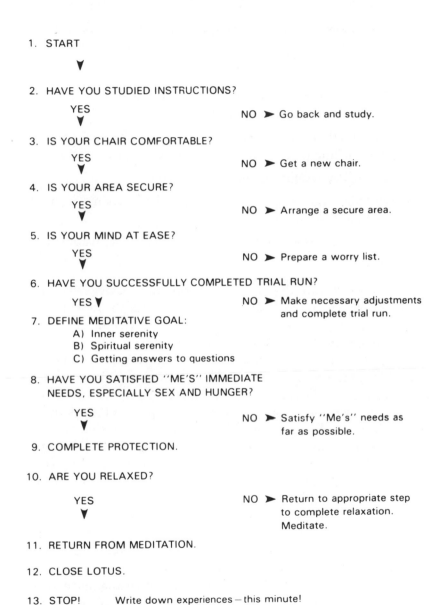

1. START
   ▼

2. HAVE YOU STUDIED INSTRUCTIONS?
        YES   NO ➤ Go back and study.
         ▼

3. IS YOUR CHAIR COMFORTABLE?
        YES   NO ➤ Get a new chair.
         ▼

4. IS YOUR AREA SECURE?
        YES   NO ➤ Arrange a secure area.
         ▼

5. IS YOUR MIND AT EASE?
        YES   NO ➤ Prepare a worry list.
         ▼

6. HAVE YOU SUCCESSFULLY COMPLETED TRIAL RUN?
        YES ▼   NO ➤ Make necessary adjustments
                                              and complete trial run.
7. DEFINE MEDITATIVE GOAL:
        A) Inner serenity
        B) Spiritual serenity
        C) Getting answers to questions

8. HAVE YOU SATISFIED "ME'S" IMMEDIATE
   NEEDS, ESPECIALLY SEX AND HUNGER?
        YES   NO ➤ Satisfy "Me's" needs as
         ▼   far as possible.

9. COMPLETE PROTECTION.

10. ARE YOU RELAXED?
        YES   NO ➤ Return to appropriate step
         ▼   to complete relaxation.
                                              Meditate.

11. RETURN FROM MEDITATION.

12. CLOSE LOTUS.

13. STOP!   Write down experiences – this minute!

Figure 15.   Flow chart of steps to outward meditation.

just give it time. Make sure as you go into meditation that a) your posture is comfortable; and b) your mind is free of worldly worries. Try the following steps:

1) Whatever thought comes to trouble and distract your mind, write it down on a piece of paper.

2) At meditation time, carry this worry-list to the opposite side of your dwelling place from the place where you meditate.

3) Put a heavy weight on the piece of paper.

4) Tell "Me" you will deal with the problems when you have finished meditation.

5) Proceed with the rest of the steps as you are accustomed to doing.

Now let's consider your health situation. Obviously pain will interfere with any quiet contemplation; but the more insidious feeling of poor health, which usually indicates the onset of a disease or a disease already present, will interfere with the mind. The usual sign that a disease is present is a feeling of warmth or cold in some part of the body. The situation must be corrected before your development can continue. Are you overtired? You must be alert but relaxed. Going to sleep is not working at development. Are you hungry? If you are starving, that fact will be uppermost in your mind and no message can get through. Similarly, if you are satiated you are just asking for trouble. Keep the body well in balance, satisfied and at peace. Then you will be able to meditate.

The human mind is an excellent unconscious detector of magnetic fields. The influence of fields can be disturbing, even fields induced by ordinary house current. Dr. Rocard of the Sorbonne has found that humans and animals can detect extremely weak fields. We have learned that even a magnetized hairpin can significantly interfere with reception of messages.

Is the lighting bothering you? It's good to work with closed eyes, though some people like to keep their eyes open and sit

with a dim red or blue or white light. It is often worthwhile
trying a change of this sort. Remember, though, that colors have
mental associations and a pale yellow candle flame is still the
best for high-level reception.

Still can't get comfortable? Knots and bindings tend to stop
the free flow of energy, and are to be avoided. Among female
meditators you usually see free-flowing hair instead of elaborate
coiffures.

Always meditate at the same time to the minute. Like you,
spirits and Guides are busy on their own assignments. If you
aren't there to keep your appointment, they become frustrated.
If you know that you won't be present next time, let them know
before you close down the previous meditation period.

The moon may also affect you. Soon you will observe the
correlation between the phases of the moon and your results.
During a waxing moon, results are more cohesive; they are
complete; the whole story is given. During a waning moon
results may be fragmentary and incomplete. You try to complete
the story—and the whole is distorted by subconscious interpretation. Reduce the overwhelming volume of complete messages
during the waxing phase by consciously rejecting those that are
negative and those that you cannot follow through on. And
know that on the waning moon you may not get the complete
picture.

If none of these things seems to be your problem, have a
glass of wine before starting; or take a vacation for a couple of
weeks. Go to a quiet mountain retreat. Relax; go out and meditate under the trees. Things will right themselves.

Now we have cautioned you, warned you, told you all the
pitfalls. Let's be optimistic for a moment and say that it is a rare
person indeed who is so scared of the images or messages, or so
turned off, that he or she will not immediately begin receiving
under much less than the ideal conditions described above. The
only requirement is practice. Do it until it becomes as natural as
washing your hands. There are no strange or exotic motions to

go through; just protect yourself and relax. If Grandpa did it following the mule, you can do it too.

As you work at meditation, you will receive a growing number of impressions through dreams and daydreams, as well as during your meditation. The impressions come into some low level of the awareness, and the conscious mind puts its own interpretation on them before they are presented to you. In this filtering, some information may be changed or lost.

As your skill in communicating grows, you will become aware of presences around you. Soon you will recognize one particular presence that visits you again and again. This is your Guide. Ask his or her name, or choose a name that feels as if it fits; when you need guidance, ask this entity for it.

When you have established communication with your Guide, he or she will tell you when you are developed enough to dispense with the salt circle. The Guide knows, so follow the advice you are given. Then you can move on and meditate for a 32-minute period, as we say, "with seed"; that is, asking questions and receiving answers.

STORE: 0286   REG: 05/01   TRAN#: 1080
SALE   04/02/1999   EMP: 00368

TANTRIC YOGA
     0343031 QP T   14.95

              Subtotal   14.95
              OHIO 7%   1.05
              Total   16.00
              CASH   20.00
              CASH   4.00-

        04/02/1999 02:50PM

THANK YOU FOR SHOPPING AT BORDERS
PLEASE ASK ABOUT OUR SPECIAL EVENTS

BORDERS

- Returns must be accompanied by receipt
- Returns must be completed within 30 days
- Merchandise must be in salable condition
- Opened videos, discs, and cassettes may be exchanged for replacement copies of the original item only
- Periodicals and newspapers may not be returned

BORDERS®

- Returns must be accompanied by receipt
- Returns must be completed within 30 days
- Merchandise must be in salable condition
- Opened videos, discs, and cassettes may be exchanged for replacement copies of the original item only
- Periodicals and newspapers may not be returned

BORDERS®

- Returns must be accompanied by receipt
- Returns must be completed within 30 days
- Merchandise must be in salable condition
- Opened videos, discs, and cassettes may b

CHAPTER
FIVE

Purification and Control

IT IS UNIVERSALLY realized that when people work in groups they must be squeaky-clean. Thus various disciplines of purification have been invented and taboos established so that the God or its image may not be defiled by unclean hands. The most extensive of these purification systems comes from the Tantrists, for the God-ess embodied in the yogi and the yogin must never be unclean. We believe that purification for the God-ess was just a method of formalizing hygienic procedures and cleanliness. It is probable that very early on, people noticed that disease and uncleanliness went together. The God-ess was thought to be showing displeasure at filth by visiting disease on the people. In modern groups aware of hygiene, however, there is no need to invoke the idea of the God-ess to justify the need for cleanliness. In selecting purifications for your own group, consider two factors:

1) the time you can allot to the purifications each day;

2) the acceptance of the purification system by members of the group.

When the group has selected the appropriate purifications, string them together into a cohesive ritual. If all members perform the same sequence each day, pretty soon the exercises become second nature. Then instead of feeling "strange" and

Table 4. Purifications

Fire	Earth	Air	Water	Exteriorization
Third Eye	Mouth	Lungs	Throat	Mind
Mouth	Intestine	Nose	Eyes	Intestine
Intestine		Intestine	Ears	
Spine			Nose	
Throat			Intestine	
Nostrils			Lingam, Yoni	
			Anus	

"different," they are comfortable, and if omitted the exercises are missed.

TYPES OF PURIFICATION

Five methods of purification are used in Tantra. They are:

1) by air;

2) by water;

3) by fire;

4) by earth;

5) by externalization.

Each part of the body—internally and externally—can be purified by any of the following techniques, but common usage has reduced the number of techniques for any given part of the body to those shown in Table 4. Let us take each body part in turn and see how the various techniques are applied.

AIR PURIFICATION

The best-known air purifying method is Yogic breathing. The ha-tha system is a 1-4-2 count breathing system designed completely to fill and (perhaps more important) completely empty the lungs. At no time should the breath be taken so rapidly that the air being drawn in or expelled will move a piece of cotton held one inch from the nostrils. Despite the hisses, grunts, and groans of many ha-tha practitioners, the original writings state clearly that the breath should not be audible. When you first start these deep-breathing exercises, you may find you are hyperventilating—getting too much oxygen into the blood. Euphoria is produced by this excess of oxygen. Some teachers of the system seem not to understand that this poisoning euphoria is not the point behind the system. If you feel dizzy, breathless, or euphoric, stop the exercise. In the first week of exercise you should take no more than four purifying breaths in any hour. We recommend you keep a brown paper grocery sack handy. If you hyperventilate, put it over your head. You may gradually increase the number of breaths as you progress, though the limit is one hundred breaths in a day or ten in any hour.

Practice now. Breathe in as deeply as you can, counting slowly as you do it. In your counting system you may need up to a count of five to breathe in completely. Now hold that breath for four times the length of time you needed to inhale; that is, if you needed five counts to inhale, hold it for twenty counts. In holding the breath, the technique is to hold the chest muscles expanded and the diaphragm relaxed. You must not stop your throat to hold your breath; instead, use your muscles. After the twenty counts, slowly and silently expel the breath until you think you have completely deflated the lungs. This should take twice the time you needed to breathe in. You will find that when your lungs feel emptied, with a little sudden push you can get a considerable amount more residual air out of the lungs. Some people lean forward so that the chest touches their knees; others place their hands on their stomach and press inward and upward. Both methods are physical aids which should be dispensed with as soon as possible. You should be able to expel the last bit of breath with a conscious contraction of your muscles and raising of your diaphragm. This is the point at which the ha-tha yoga people tell you to go "tha!" but in Tantra silence is maintained.

If you do deep breathing during a sunrise ritual, it is pleasant to help your partner expel the last breath by placing your hands below the diaphragm and pressing hard. Usually only one or two purification breaths are taken during a sunrise ritual.

If you enjoy walking, purification breathing can be fitted naturally into your walking stride. You can also use it at the beginning of one-pointed meditation. The subtle difference between the active purification breathing and the passive or meditative breathing is the length of the cycle. The body needs more oxygen when you are walking than it does when you are sitting in meditation; consequently the breathing cycle in meditation becomes very long. In meditation some yogis take one breath a minute. Others have learned to control their breathing to such an extent that they need less than one breath an hour. The more you practice purification breathing, the better will be your health and your control over your body.

Through purification breathing, Komar, who in "real" life is a cheese maker from Wooster, Ohio, is able to control physical pain to such an extent that he can walk on fire, lie on beds of nails while heavy weights are placed on him, and literally be crucified by having nails driven into his hands. Not only does he feel no pain, but when the nails are removed he does not bleed!

Cleansing the Bowels with Air

The next stage of air purification is purification of bowels and the digestive tract. In the West, belching and farting are considered antisocial behavior; but in the East, it is realized that retaining gases within the body is dangerous. To dilute the gases and to bring them out more readily, air is swallowed and added to the normal production of intestinal gases. The "crow mouth" system is used. The lips are pursed into something resembling the beak of a crow. The mouth is filled with little sips of air and this air is consciously swallowed, until the stomach is noticeably expanded with the air. When the stomach is expanded, the hands are used in a firm massaging action for as long as five minutes to press the stomach downward and push the air into the intestines. When the massage is complete, the worker lies flat on the floor until the air is naturally expelled either in belching or through the anus. If a large belch results, on the next occasion more time is spent in trying to massage the air downward into the lower intestinal tract, for belching is not the object of the exercise. The object is to make sure the air passes completely through the intestine.

Cleansing the Nose with Air

Nose-cleansing is done by using the normal purification breathing, but closing off one nostril for the inhaling breath and the other nostril for the exhaling breath.

WATER PURIFICATION

The first purification by water is external. Every body part is washed with soap and hot water, then carefully re-washed in cool clean water. This is a twice-daily complete washing. It is often followed by complete immersion, the head and everything else going under the water. Today's popular hot tubs are ideally suited to this type of immersion and soaking. In cleaning the hands, the nails are carefully cleansed and are kept quite short. The hands are always washed last, after the very careful washing of the genitalia. It is very nice to have bidets in the bathroom. All salt water solutions in the following purifications are made by mixing one teaspoon of salt into one cup of warm water. You can double or triple these amounts if more water is called for.

Purification of the Lingam and the
Yoni by Water

In washing the lingam, a soft rubber ear-syringe is used to inject salt water solution very gently into the urethra. This is the last act before copulation and is obviously designed to make sure that no bacteria are carried into the yoni. For the female, the external parts of the yoni are carefully cleansed but internal douching is not generally used because semen is a natural antibiotic; and if it remains in the yoni and is allowed to be expelled naturally the yoni remains healthy. Of course occasionally the females will want to douche. When they do, the internal surfaces of the yoni should be relubricated before copulation. In lieu of the commercial douches used by many females, we recommend that you use a vinegar and water douche, adding 1/4 cup vinegar to 2 cups of lukewarm water.

Purification of the Nose by Water

The nose and nasal passages are purified by sniffing up salt water. Each nostril in turn should be immersed and about one tablespoon of salt water sucked into the nostril. The water is then expelled by blowing out, although some of it may be swallowed. The use of strings through the nostrils as recommended in old texts is to be avoided.

Purification of the Throat by Water

The purification of the throat by water is done by gargling salt water. This is not the hearty, noisy gargle commonly practiced by Westerners. It is a soft, gentle expulsion of one inhaled breath through water held in the gullet with the head thrown back, then spitting the water out.

Purification of the Mouth by Water

Normal Western toothbrushing is used; purists replace the toothbrush with a piece of acacia root. After the teeth are thoroughly cleansed, they are picked with a piece of acacia wood passed between the teeth. (Modern dental floss is an acceptable substitute for this step.)

Purification of the Ears by Water

The ears are now cleansed with water, using the same soft rubber syringe as for the lingam. Salt water is used by many; others prefer a weak solution of hydrogen peroxide.[1]

Purification of the Intestines by Water

The last of the morning water purifications is the drinking of at least two full cups (one pint) of cool water. This may be sipped slowly while you enjoy the warm water of a hot tub.

Purification of the Eyes by Water

This is done with natural tears. Everyone in the house must weep at least once a day: not from sorrow but to cleanse the eyes. Sitting perhaps in the hot tub, gaze at a small object about ten feet away that is about the size of a silver dollar. The object must be large enough to be seen easily but not large enough so the eyes must move to view it comfortably. The gaze is maintained unblinking until the eyes water and cry. In a hot tub of reasonable size, the aureole of a breast (male or female) can serve as the object of such concentrated gaze.

Purification of the Anus by Water

This morning purification is considered by old-line Tantrists to be one of the most important parts of the purification ritual. Many spiritualists have followed this practice. The high colonics of the followers of Edgar Cayce are but one example of a spiritual sect that places much reliance for spiritual growth on this one exercise. To modern Tantrists, such a fixation seems a little extreme; perhaps you should have your group try it for at least a

---

[1]One tablespoonful to a cup of water.

month and see whether your experience bears out that of the rest of the world in deciding on its efficacy as a pathway toward spiritual development.

The simple pressure douche bags traditionally used by women may be used for these enemas (for that is the essence of the treatment). About two cups of warm salted water is used for the injection. The mixture is usually made by placing salt in the douche bag before filling it under pressure at the tap. Needless to say, the enema is given while you sit on the toilet. Any female will be able to instruct the males in the use of the equipment. The insertion wands and douche bags used for enemas should be kept carefully separate from those which the women use for vaginal douching.

When the enema is not used, an acceptable water purification of the posterior yoni is achieved by standing in water up to the navel and rapidly squatting several times.

FIRE PURIFICATION

Tantrists are sun worshippers by nature. Part of every day is given over to purification of the body by the fiery rays of the sun. It is considered that the hands and face receive sufficient sunlight from normal everyday activities; though, of course, if you are largely confined to indoors this is not necessarily true. The area of concentration is the back and front of the torso, including the stomach and the lingam. Normal sunlamp regimens may be used in accordance with the manufacturer's recommended schedules, not to maintain a tan in the cosmetic sense, but just a healthy vigor. In addition to the normal manufacturer's warnings about eye damage, we say again: be very, very careful about exposing eyes, face, or the backs of your hands to sunlamps. Any time your eyes feel dry or the least bit prickly, make sure that your goggles are properly fitted and have no pinholes. Any reddening of the skin is a signal to reduce exposure time. Real sun is better for your body if you live in a climate where you see it!

Purification of the Mouth by Fire

The gums are energetically rubbed at least once a week with baking soda. On other days the gums are gently rubbed with clean earth or with a little salt. Next a small piece of flat wood is used to scrape the upper surface of the tongue. Though this step sounds distressing, in fact it is pleasant and gives the tongue a very good morning feel, as well as preventing bad breath. After scraping, the tongue is rubbed with a speck of peppermint-flavored butter.[2] Only a tiny dab is needed to make your tongue feel glowing and alive. In the morning a mouthful of smoke (hot air) from the first fire lighted is gulped in and expelled.

Purification of the Belly by Fire

Lying on your back, apply pressure to the navel so that it is pushed backward and upward toward the spine. Form a fist of your right hand and clasp it within your left hand. Press the fist into the navel and pull the navel up and toward the spine. On a normal morning, five such pulls are recommended. When you have time—for instance on a weekend—100 pulls are beneficial. As you rise from this purification, try to hold your stomach muscles so that the navel remains in the up-and-back position. As weeks and months go by, you will find it gradually becomes easier and easier for the stomach muscles to hold this position. The purification by fire tremendously improves the posture of anyone who has any belly flab.

Purification of the Intestines by Fire

Lie on your back and vigorously shove the belly from one side to the other. On normal mornings ten or fifteen such back-and-forth motions should be done; but on unscheduled days, 100 are

---

[2]Steep fresh mint leaves in melted butter for a half-hour; then strain.

prescribed. Together with the enema, the exercises for the stomach and the intestines provide a digestive benefit which Westerners have not yet understood.

Purification of the Spinal Column by Fire

This is a scraping of the spinal column by your dyadic partner. Tradition prescribes that it be scraped with a stone or a shell; however, we find that the old fashioned loofah sponge works the best. This is not a harsh scraping but the gentle removal of dead skin and cells that accumulate during the day. One or two strokes from the hairline all the way down the spine, done slowly but firmly, are the approved method. This oily area of the body cannot easily be reached by its owner. Many Tantrists use a little flowing water during this purification; but if the loofah is occasionally dipped in water, this is not really essential.

Other Purifications by Fire

Two fire-purification methods popular in India may not be adaptable to your group, but we are including them in case some of you might be interested.

Throat Cleansing: A piece of soft cotton cloth about two inches wide and nine inches long is moistened in salt water. It is swallowed until just the very end of it is left outside the lips; then it is pulled out and thrown away. (It may be laundered and disinfected for reuse.) This procedure removes all the phlegm in the throat and eliminates those nasty sore throats that occur so often in the autumn.

Cleansing of the throat can also be done with the internal soft part of a palm tree. A beeswax candle has come to be the accepted instrument since parts of palm trees are not available to most Western Tantrists. The procedure is to tilt the head well back, insert the stick about one inch into the gullet, and withdraw it. Apparently this practice is just as beneficial as the cloth-swallowing system. It is obvious that many circus performers employ Tantric techniques of cloth-swallowing and stick-swallowing to perform their razor blade and sword-swallowing acts.

Nostril Cleansing: A small piece of string about twelve inches long is sniffed up the nostril and hacked forward onto the tongue and pulled out of the mouth. A small knot is tied in the end and the knot is pulled through the nostril and out the mouth. We do not recommend that anyone use this procedure; it is included here only for information.

EARTH PURIFICATION

The earth purifications are done to bring us back to the realization of our dependence on the products of the earth. Tantrists regard them as balancing elements in life. Earth purification gets us back in touch with the source of our life and its pleasures. When someone is completely adrift in the spiritual world, the mundane is brought back with earth purifications. All is a balance: fire, earth, air, water. Without any one of these, the practitioner loses spiritual balance and becomes less well directed.

Purification of the Intestines by Earth

This is currently interpreted to mean eating nuts and unprocessed grains and seeds, bran-type cereals, and all the coarse, dry, sugarless cereals available today. In the old days, eating clean earth was also recommended. Despite quite a lot of research, we have not been able clearly to define what "clean earth" is, so we cannot tell you what to eat for it.

Sometimes eating cereals, especially unprocessed ones, during the gourmet banquet is a sign that the person is constipated or in need of earth purification.

Purification of the Forehead by Fire

The last and perhaps most important fire purification area is the forehead. Again this is done by one-half of a dyadic pair to the partner. First the skin across the brows is gently oiled and pushed toward the center and slightly upward. Then the very center of the forehead between the eyes is massaged with a little oil or peppermint butter. The massaging partner exerts as much weight as can easily be borne, then washes the area with a soapy cloth. In the house the red dot of purification is then applied.

PURIFICATION BY EXTERIORIZATION

To put it plainly, this system is alien to Western minds. The first part is easy, but the second part (often done simultaneously with the first by Indian Tantrists) should not be even attempted by Westerners.

Exteriorization of the Head

This is done by simply thinking of those pressing problems you have, writing them down in a list, and taking them away from the ritual area. This gets your problems out on paper and allows you to lay them aside while you continue your rituals. You say to yourself, "I will deal with those problems at such-and-such a time. Right now I'm going to work my rituals." This is a simple exteriorization of thoughts, an extremely healthful and positive process, especially when you can share your problems with the other members of a group; for all burdens are made lighter by sharing.

Exteriorization of the Intestine

In conjunction with mental exteriorization an Indian Tantrist pulls part of the large intestine out through the anus. This is the exteriorization of the bowel. It is washed and then sucked back inside. This is technically a prolapse of the rectum. Under no circumstances should you follow the Indian mystic's path of exteriorizing thoughts and bowel at the same time. Thoughts, yes; bowel, no.

A method of posterior exteriorizing that can safely be used in the West is as follows: Sit on the floor with two small blocks of wood, one under each buttock. Spread your legs slightly and stretch them out before you. Bend forward until your forehead comes as close to the floor as possible. Grasp the backs of your calves. Slowly and rhythmically open and close the sphincter muscles. Synchronize this with the exteriorization of mental problems you may have.

LIMBERING EXERCISES

Tantric exercise is designed to limber the body, stretch the muscles, and improve flexibility and adaptability of the muscles and joints. The idea is not to turn the student into a superman or -woman. Great bunches of knotted muscles are unsightly to the Tantrist. A smooth, supple body with hidden internal reserves and strength is the aim. Any time you sweat, pant, or in any way get overheated, you should stop the exercise; for panting, sweating, and overheating are all considered to be signs that you are drawing on your reserves. You are not to draw on your reserves during exercise — only when they are needed in emergencies. As you follow the exercise pattern you will find you can do more and more each day with less effort. You can stretch further, you can open your legs wider, you can bend your back more easily, and your neck especially becomes more supple.

As with many Tantric practices, when the exercises are put together into a series, confusion is replaced with order and the order brings with it enlightenment. Any time exercises become a drudgery, drop them from your schedule.

Exercises are usually carried out in pairs. If a dyadic couple is severely mismatched in weight or size, however, it is permissible just for the exercise period to change partners. This is not a recommended practice but one which makes obvious sense.

The Tantric exercises are usually taken from the general Hatha Yoga practice; but here they are adapted for work in couples, emphasizing muscles that will be used in ritual. In all the exercises, continuous, deep, slow breathing is important. Ha-tha breaths are often used, one per exercise cycle. Under no circumstances should you strain by stopping breathing during exercise; that is, don't hold your breath.

A very basic exercise is the pelvic tilt, designed to develop control of the lingam and the yoni and to strengthen the thrusting muscles in the small of the back and in the stomach. When the females recognize the advantage of being able to adjust the position of the clitoris against the lingam, they really enjoy this exercise.

Basic Exercise

This is done sitting in the sunrise ritual position with the lingam in the yoni. The female sits upright with her back perfectly straight. She leans slightly forward and puts her hands on her thighs. She tilts her pelvis so that the labia and the clitoris are rubbed along the centerline of the male's abdomen. She tries to get the maximum tilting motion. This means that she tries to reach as high up the male's abdomen with the clitoris as possible; then she tilts to reach as high as possible on the lingam while maintaining pelvic contact. (A minimum of eight rotations should be done in each cycle.) Then she lies forward on the male while he tilts his pelvis so that the lingam alternately reaches high inside the yoni and is almost completely extracted from the yoni. As he learns to tilt the pelvis more, the female must lift herself up from him because he will be able to remove the lingam completely from the yoni in the downward tilt, interrupting the exercise.

The Rising Sun and Moon

This exercise combines the pelvic thrust with strengthening of the female's pectoral muscles. Standing to face the male, the female places her hands behind his neck, then grips her right forearm with her left hand and her left forearm with her right hand. He puts his hands on her hips and brings his belly into firm contact with hers. Her nipples should be just touching his chest. She tenses her arm muscles and her pectorals to lift the breasts, and rubs the nipples across his chest. At the same time he tenses his stomach muscles, pulling his stomach in and the lingam upward. While they do this, the partners look intently into each other's eyes. Each partner does at least 8 contractions; 32 are the full practice.

The Closing of the Arch

This exercise uses a silver dollar. While the Tantrist stands upright, the silver dollar is pressed between the buttocks just above the posterior yoni and the muscles hold it in position. The dyadic partner gently strokes the stomach very lightly with the fingertips until slight muscular tremors are felt, then stops. This exercise develops muscle control.

The Eclipse

The male stands facing the female. Each jumps to open their feet to the fullest extent, simultaneously raising their arms over their head and clapping their hands. (The male's right hand claps the female's left hand and vice versa.) The jump is repeated, bringing the feet together, and the hands swing down to clap the thighs. Both partners then come up onto their toes and stretch high while gradually bringing their hands to the full outward position above their heads with palms up. They hold this position for a moment and then come down to a flat-footed position, bring their arms down, and begin a slow knee bend. The knees must be opened slightly so that one knee can go between the partner's legs. They go down until their knuckles just touch the floor, then they slowly stand again. This exercise is done slowly while partners maintain full eye contact. Eight cycles are usually prescribed.

The Cobra and the Swan

The female lies on the floor on her back with her legs straight out, as wide apart as possible. The male holds her ankles and moves her legs a little wider apart. (When you first start this exercise you will be surprised at how much further apart the legs will progressively move as the days go by.) The male then lies between her legs and the lingam is inserted into the yoni (this is optional). He puts his hands on the floor under her armpits and lifts himself up, maintaining pelvic contact. This is the Cobra. As he lifts, the female pushes upward with the tips of both fingers on the sides of his jaw. She must be careful not to lift too hard, especially the first time the exercise is done. Both relax their arms and then stretch upward again. Eight cycles are recommended in this position. The female closes her legs under the male. If the partners are coupled, they try to remain so while they roll over. The male spreads his legs as wide as possible. The female lets her knees come down onto the floor. The male holds her arms very close to her shoulders and lifts her off himself. She spreads her arms out and as far back as she can, gracefully pulling her head back with chin out and arms back, going into Swan posture. Again pelvic contact is maintained. As a last move in this exercise, some females are able to lift their breasts with their pectoral muscles. The posture is held for one complete breath. Then it is repeated for a total of 4 times. At the end of the cycle the female kneels backward between the male's legs and pushes his feet apart. The male pelvis is less flexible than the female, so this exercise is even more important for the male than for the female and she should be rather firm with him.

The Rocking Chair

The dyad sit on the floor facing each other with the male's feet under the female's buttocks, knees together. Her legs go outside his and tuck under his upper thighs or buttocks. Each lies back to reach a position flat on the floor. They sit up, the slower the better. At first it may be necessary for them to use their hands to help themselves up; later they will be able to sit up slowly without using their hands. When they are vertical they stretch their hands out to each side and then bring them up over their heads and grasp them together. This is a strenuous exercise, yet it is still recommended. Eventually you will be able to complete eight cycles without strain.

The Bow

Another exercise for back flexibility is done by lying on the stomach and reaching backward to grasp your ankles. When you have your ankles, move your head slowly backward and rock gently on the stomach. If you cannot start this motion, your partner should rock you four or five times back and forth quite slowly from the knees to the chin.

The Arch

This exercise is the reverse of the Bow, in that you lie flat on your back and arch the small of your back away from the floor. It is easiest to put the feet against a wall and with the hands flat on the floor gently inch yourself toward the wall, arching the stomach upward. Four repetitions of this exercise are recommended.

Riding

This benefits the male pelvic area. The male lies flat on his stomach. The female sits on his buttocks with knees on the floor and toes hooked over the top of his knees. He lifts her by lifting his pelvis clear of the floor. The slower the lift and the longer the hold, the better. Four complete cycles of this exercise should be accomplished.

The Sunflower

It is often said that you are as young as your neck. There are four distinct exercises specifically for the neck that you do facing your partner. If you can make your partner smile or laugh, so much the better.

In all the neck exercises, never go to the pain level at any time, and do not jerk or try to crack any vertebrae. In this exercise, you nod, alternately burying your chin in your chest and lifting the chin as high as possible. Do not jerk at the end of the cycle; instead make it a smooth, slow nod. Then look as far as you can to the right and as far as you can to the left. Roll your head slowly around in a circular motion. Lay your head down on your right shoulder and then on your left shoulder so your ear tries to touch the shoulder. Eighteen of each of these motions are recommended.

The Ostrich

Commonly all Tantra yogis have been trained from a young age to stand on their head for eight minutes a day. People coming to Tantra later in life, however, have difficulty doing this exercise. The important thing is to get the head below the pelvis. This can be done in many ways. Let us consider first a kneeling ostrich. Place both hands on the floor so that when you put your head down the top of the head will be cradled by your hands. In the kneeling posture, put your head on the floor.

For the full Ostrich, get your dyadic partner to help you stand on your head. Maintain this position for eight minutes. If you experience any dizziness when you first put your head down or when you sit up, do not continue the exercise. Instead have your blood pressure checked. If the blood pressure is normal but you still have dizziness, you should avoid doing the exercise.

The Gargoyle

This is sometimes called "lion face." These exercises teach control of the facial muscles so you reveal emotions only when you want to. The exercises also remove wrinkles and keep the tone of the facial muscles so your face doesn't droop with age:

Tongue: Push your tongue out of your mouth and try to touch the tip of your nose with it. Then move your jaw to one side and then to the other (with the tongue out). Let the tongue return and repeat the jaw exercise.

Cheek Muscles and Lips: Pull your lips into a snarl; then open your mouth and pull the upper lip down as far as possible over the front teeth. Many more facial exercises can be done. If you do those we have listed, your face will remain young and flexible.

Eyes: Eye exercises fall into several categories. Cross-gender palmings are very beneficial for someone who wears glasses. If you have a large group, a circle is formed, Indian-file. The hands from the person behind are placed over the eyes of the person before. The circle remains stationary while each worker concentrates on healing the eyes of the person in front of him or her. After eight Ha-tha breaths, reverse directions and palm the eyes of the person who previously palmed yours. Again eight ha-tha breaths are taken. If only a dyad is working, they palm each other's eyes while facing each other; then each faces away in turn to have his or her eyes palmed with the opposite hand. In other words, the right hand goes to the right eye and the left hand goes to the left eye when they are both facing in the same direction, and the right hand goes to the left eye and the left hand to the right eye when they face each other.

The second eye exercise requires a bright light. The intensity of the light and your distance from it should be arranged so that the eye does not hurt when you look steadily at the light. Switch the light on, and gaze at it for the duration of one breath. Switch the light off and wait for two breaths. Repeat the cycle a total of four times.

Probably the most important single eye exercise is for depth of vision. Here you stretch both hands out in front of you, palms upward. Put your middle finger up. Gradually bring both middle fingers in toward the eyes. Try to keep the eyes in focus as you bring the fingers in. This should be slowly repeated for a total of eight cycles.

To develop peripheral vision stretch your hands out in front, palms up, the middle fingers up. Swing your arms slowly outward to each side. Gazing directly ahead, see how far you can move your arms outward without losing sight of your fingers. Eight cycles are recommended.

Eye-widening and -slitting: Pull the forehead up and the cheeks down to make the eyes widen. Pull the eyebrows down hard and the cheeks up to make the eyes slit. These two exercises help with forehead wrinkles as well as with the smile-wrinkles in the corners of the eyes ("crow's feet").

COMBINATION EXERCISES

Combination exercises with the group are always more enjoyable than those done alone or even in dyad. A typical traditional bridge/stretching exercise follows.

Stand with your back to your partner, tops of your heads touching. Gradually move your feet outward and arch your back so that a space is developed between the two backs sufficient for a person to pass through. You may find that you must hold your hands above your head to maintain balance. Starting with all members of the house back to back facing outward, alternating male and female, the end couple breaks the position and forces itself through the tunnel. Then they take up their position at the end of the tunnel. When all dyads have passed through the tunnel, the exercise is complete.

Wheelbarrow races, tippy-toe, three-legged walks—many playful exercises are very good for you and can be fun, especially if some simple forfeits are added to the game. When people from different houses meet, sometimes a large ring is suspended and a competition held as to who can make the worst face simply by using facial muscles without any help from hands or fingers.

It is usual to spend lots of time in the exercise room on the weekend or when the general schedule is relaxed. Be inventive. Remember that the exercises are designed for gentle stretching and compression of the muscles. Holding the posture for a full ha-tha breath is more important than working up a sweat.

CHAPTER
SIX

Cycles of Sex, Food, and Work

TANTRISTS LIVE THEIR lives by a different clock than do other people. They live by the cycles of the heavens, specifically the cycles of the moon as it waxes and wanes, and the cycles of the sun as its motion alternates between winter cold and summer heat. It is the interlacing of the moon cycle and the sun cycle with the rosters of work and ritual that makes the overlapping phases of Tantric life always interesting, always changeable, always well worth living. The Tantrist never wakes up to just another day; for each day new and natural heavenly changes occur, and as growth progresses, so the cycles move from chaos through order to internal acceptance, understanding, and development. Balancing these daily changes is the firm foundation of the unchanging rituals of exercise and work. Any time the Tantrist feels unsure, he or she is reassured by this—the never-changing part of life. Partners may change, work assignments may change, but the ritual remains unchanged as it has for untold centuries.

From the Tantrist's viewpoint, the key to understanding the month lies in the chakras and the symbols shown in Table 2 (see page 44). As the month progresses, each few days you enter into a time of changed feelings. The transition is not sudden or abrupt, but slow and cyclical. Four red petals become six vermilion tears. You climb from animalistic lustful behavior toward

controlled spiritual behavior as the amount of sexual contact
increases or decreases and the drives rhythmically change.

FUTURE SERENITY

Start working today toward the serene future. Many of the ideas
in the following pages describe an ideal situation: a light at the
end of a tunnel, a situation toward which you should strive.
Always proceed with happiness and joy. Do not make the
attainment of the goal such a grim assignment as to detract from
the exquisite pleasure of trying. Though your paycheck job may
interfere with the attainment of the blessed moon cycle, though
your life partner may be too uptight sexually for you to change
partners or even achieve regular climaxes, slowly and gradually
bring changes into your life until you can achieve your goals.
Don't hold out for perfection, doing nothing until every tiniest
stipulation is fulfilled. The longest journey begins with a single
step. Take that single step today; otherwise you will still be
waiting to start as you are carted away to the boneyard.

THE HEAVENLY CYCLE

The very basis of life on this planet is controlled by the moon
and the sun. The sun controls the Mother's annual cycle of
birth, growth, and death. Natural births and deaths, menstruation, the tides in the ocean and in our bodily emotional cycles,
are all controlled by the moon. Accidents, emotional instability,
and bodily bloating all occur at full moon. Therefore Tantrists
arrange their work life so that little work is done and little food
is eaten at full moon. Instead, at this time emotions are given full
range. Naturally if you are working in the outside world, this
cannot always be arranged; but if possible, you should work less

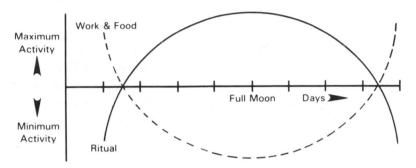

Figure 16.   Cycles of work and ritual.

overtime or at less strenuous tasks at full moon than you do at new moon. It is also true that skilled work (especially with cutting tools) goes much better at new moon that it does at full moon. In a local furniture-crafting factory they do all the lathe and cutting work at new moon and all the fine sanding and polishing at full moon. They simply have fewer accidents this way.

It is important for the yogins to arrange their menstrual period so that it coincides with new moon. In this way there will be a minimum of bloating during menstruation and they will be able to participate in the Kundalini Ritual.[1]

The spiritual moon cycle, sometimes called the ritual cycle, peaks as the moon approaches full, when all members of the

---

[1]The cycle can be adjusted through limited use of the pill, but in most houses the females synchronize to one another after a month or two—a well-known Tantric phenomenon but one that has only recently been "discovered" by Western researchers in women's dorms and nurses' quarters.

house attempt the Kundalini Ritual. The sexual cycle, therefore, goes from a minimum of ritual activity to a maximum as the work cycle does the opposite. This pattern is shown in figure 16. Notice particularly that the cycles lag behind the moon phase by four days. The maximum food intake of the cycle corresponds to the maximum work and minimum sexual activity at new moon, and maximum sexual activity coincides with the maximum ritual activity and minimum food intake at full moon.

Tantrists live their religion every day of their lives. They don't just go to a special place one day a week. So the spiritual cycle builds gradually to a peak and then gradually comes down to the minimum. There are no sudden changes and no surprises. Many people seem to think that after a time of heavy sexual activity there should be a sudden stop—a recovery period; but in a situation where stimulation is high, the body adapts to the high performance level and problems (both emotional and physical) occur only if "cold turkey" withdrawal is attempted.

WARNING

You will find that far from lowering the need for orgasms, the training increases the need. A Western wife may often say to her husband, "You've had enough. We did it last night." The Tantrists realize that as sexual activity increases and hormone levels change, so more is needed and sex must be tapered off, never suddenly stopped. Tantric gurus warn people that they should not enter into this discipline and expect to be able to leave in the middle of a month. They talk of madness and hysteria resulting if you do try to leave a Tantra house except during the dark of the moon. This is simply the result of the body's adjustment to the high sexual hormone levels. It is as if you tried to stop smoking or drinking coffee "cold turkey."

FOOD CYCLES

If you look at the Tantric prescribed food intake for a month, you will find they do not eat a balanced diet on a daily basis. Their intake of nutrients goes from fast to satiation. But over a month's time the diet is carefully balanced. Traditionally, the month is broken into four separate segments with respect to food:

1) For the four days before full moon, a total fast is observed. Some members may not be able to accomplish this; in their case only whole grain breads, nuts, honey, and water are consumed. Some groups include fresh green fruit in this diet. When fruit is eaten, the seeds are carefully saved and planted.

2) At full moon, red meat is added to the diet a little at a time. As the moon wanes the quantity of red meat is increased, reaching a maximum in the days before new moon. It is thought that the increase of red meat was originally designed to provide both the high energies needed for work at new moon and an ample supply of iron for the menstruating females.

3) In the four days after new moon, the meals become luxurious and of gourmet quality. At the final new moon meal marking the end of the sexual fast, each cook tries to outdo the previous one in the preparation of the most luxurious gourmet meal a house can afford. It is part of Tantric tradition that aperitifs, two wines, and a brandy accompany this meal. It starts with a fish dish, proceeds to a fowl dish, to a beef dish, and to a carameled dessert followed by cheese and fruit. This is the one meal in the month that is a real blowout in a Tantric house. It is the meal which has caused Tantrists to have the name of gluttonous sensualists; in fact stories of their rolling on the floor stuffing their mouths and pouring wine on each other are not uncommon. The whole point here is not to eat and drink until you are incapacitated or sick, but to savor a fine meal among pleasant companions, to taste each dish and relish the ingredients with

which it is made; for in the following days till full moon the taste buds will not again be thus titillated.

4) After the new moon feast, red meat is eliminated from the diet and chicken and pork are substituted. After about a week, white meats are replaced with fish. Then fish with vegetables only is eaten until the fast begins for the next full moon. This is a period of bland foods, when spices are removed from the food as the fast approaches.

Tantrists of our acquaintance have embraced the nouvelle cuisine movement originating in France, for those lightly cooked vegetables arranged in attractive patterns on the plate, the savory sauces, and a small portion of flesh are exactly what the Tantrist strives for.

THE SEXUAL MOON CYCLE

The food cycle is offset from the cycle of sexual activity by half a moon period. You can see exactly the same sensory satiation and withdrawal occurring in one as in the other. The complete cycle is shown in figure 17.

Starting four or five days before new moon, a total sexual fast is observed, during which no orgasms occur. Depending on the house and the outside work load, some rituals are still observed; for instance, if a yogin is not menstruating the lingam enters the yoni in the sun ritual but no overt sexual motions are made. This is simply the observance of a standard ritual. There is nothing more disruptive in a Tantric house than members who deliberately arouse sexual desires in one of the other gender during this period. Yes, there is still a lot of touching; yes, there is still a lot of loving behavior. Members are looking forward to the whole re-awakened cycle of orgasms; and through this postponement of present pleasure for future Nirvana they learn control.

This interlude may be viewed by outsiders as weird or deviant. Here is a whole group of people living together, continually enjoying one another—and suddenly everything is switched off. The reasoning in the minds of the Tantrists is clear: "We learn to control ourselves by this means. We go from the exquisite pleasure of the Kundalini Circle to the exquisite pleasure of living with someone, adoring this person, looking after this person—and not having orgasm. Orgasms are absolutely denied; it is a will-strengthening process that we are going through. Those who don't like our ways don't have to live by them."

The only person who will know you have had an orgasm is yourself and your partner. No one will blame you or accuse you of a great sin. You will know that next month you will do better.

During the fast period, spontaneous turn-ons may happen to both yogis and yogins, especially among young or new house members. Gradually as more skilled mental control is achieved,

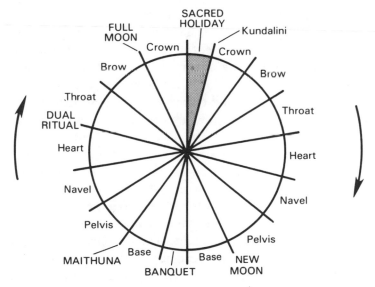

Figure 17. The tantric master cycle.

these arousals and the associated raising of erectile tissues diminish. At no time should anyone criticize one who lacks absolute control. Turn-ons are in fact a sign of beauty and sexual skill appreciated: a compliment, not an insult.

In this five-day period, dyadic couples sleep together. It is the only time during the month they are required to sleep in the same bed. There is a Tantric tradition which is also found in early European and Japanese thought: that sleeping with a partner but not having intercourse gives each partner new strength. Virgins are brought to lie with the old sick king. When Gandhi was recovering from a fast, virgins were brought to lie with him. The subtle exchange of energy is something that has to be experienced to be understood. It is the joining of the male and female principles and the willing giving of energy to one another.

Since much of the house schedule is suspended at this time, it is the time when house members take the opportunity to go out and do many of the things that are impossible when the more rigid, arduous schedule is being observed. Dyadic couples stay together during these outings. Of course people can double-date, or the whole group can go out together, but couples always stay with their partners. In the old way, when they were out of the protection of the house, the man was instructed always to stay within six feet of the woman. Here is a chance for the man to display his gallantry—not in a big macho way, by leading a female into difficulties and extracting her from them—but in a low-key way. He is protecting a most precious piece of humankind: a Tantric lady. She is irreplaceable. Of course, if the man gets into trouble, the female will also do her best to help and protect him, for he too with all his training is irreplaceable. Chivalry and gallantry are words that have their place here. There is nothing wrong with the male opening the door and seeing what is inside before the lady enters. There is nothing wrong with her preceding him into a known environment. Have fun. Be courteous. Play the Knight and the Lady.

The sexual fast ends four hours after the gourmet meal. In a typical case the meal will take place at 7 or 8 A.M. and the rite will be observed at noon as the moon crosses the zenith. This is the great Welcoming Back of the Moon Rite, the cycle of the heavens here being represented in microcosm by the Maithuna ritual. Members acknowledge in the ritual that the cycle of life is inseparable from the moon's waxing and waning. Few exercises are done on this day since it is one of the two days of contemplation during the month.

THE MAITHUNA RITUAL

The great monthly welcoming festival takes place for all members in the exercise room. It is preceded by special loving and petting. Since this is a male or new moon ritual, after the meal the male is worshipped by the female. She caresses him and does any grooming that needs doing. He is oiled and massaged and made as god-like as poor human bodies can be. All members assume the maithunic position and attempt to maintain their partners on the brink of orgasm for 32 minutes. After this period, all rise. A circle dance is started within a protective circle. The force is raised and the agreed ritual is performed. (The target for the force has been agreed by all beforehand.) Only when this ritual is complete are the dyadic couples allowed to retire for completion. The thing that drives the circle is sexual desire. If orgasms occur before the ritual itself is complete, there will be less energy because—just like the donkey and the carrot—there is nothing leading and driving the circle forward.

The Maithuna ritual requires the greatest sexual control of any ritual during the month; for no orgasms occur during the ritual, even though prolonged sexual contact is made and a great deal of loving and touching occurs. Most couples go for completion, and orgasms are encouraged as soon as possible after the closing of the ritual. The yogis make a special effort: If completion is not achieved, they may get temporary muscle spasms and cramp, though these quickly pass away.

During the eight days following the moon festival, ritual copulation occurs once a day in the evening just before sleeping. The phrase "ritual copulation" means that both partners spend eight minutes in touching where they both single-pointedly concentrate on the anticipated sex act. Then the lingam is inserted into the yoni. Each partner carefully arouses the other until both are close to orgasm, holding this state for sixteen minutes. Both partners then come quickly to orgasm and remain coupled thereafter until the tension is released (another eight minutes). This ritual copulation usually occurs in the male's sleeping area. In any case both partners return to their respective beds to sleep. It is an honor for a male to be invited to a female's room.

Following the eight days of one ritual copulation a day, the pace increases to two a day. The second encounter is usually arranged for early morning. The house is roused. Each member urinates and if possible evacuates the bowels. The lingam and yoni are washed and purified, and another ritual copulation occurs.

This is usually a slow, gentle, lethargic experience. In this moist, quiet time secret spaces are explored. It is a time for gentle whispering and touching, trying different things in different positions, total enjoyment, until after a prolonged time the deep slow orgasm is achieved. It may be, in fact, that the partners are so lethargic that they even fall asleep coupled without ever attaining orgasm. There is nothing wrong or shameful in falling asleep with your dyadic partner. The whole point is exploration, trying new things, finding out what is best for this couple to give the most exquisite, deep, mind-blowing, earth-shattering experience that stirs every part of each one's very being. Musicians talk about theme and variations. This is the time to invent variations. If you want to invite another couple to the play, bring them. Usually the sleeping rooms are not suitable for group work, so you can move more comfortably to the exercise room. There are no prohibitions. The two-a-day pace continues for eight days in the middle of the cycle.

THE KUNDALINI CIRCLE

Four days after full moon at the end of the food fast, an entire day is devoted to the performance of the great Kundalini Circle rite. In the great full moon female festival, the goddess is worshipped in her incarnation as woman. Activity starts in the exercise room. The males are totally subservient to the females. Any grooming the yogins want, they get. Any little services they want doing, they get. They are worshipped, massaged, oiled, and petted. At the prescribed time the cycle of the ritual begins. Each of the four phases takes 32 minutes. The phases are:

Eating: Green grapes or another green fruit, white cheese, water, and nuts are taken, together with tiny portions of cold beef, fish, and fowl. These tiny portions are no bigger than that which will cover a thumbnail. They are not intended for nourishment; they are intended just to remind the practitioners of the foods they eat during the month.

Washing and Purification: This is a standard exercise, the same as you do each morning.

Ritual Copulation: Some Tantric houses insist this must be done in public in full view of one another and timed so that as many orgasms as possible occur exactly at the end of 32 minutes; other houses prefer the privacy of the sleeping quarters.

Resting and Meditation: The partners stay together in the same bed and rest for 16 minutes. After that each meditates for 16 minutes.

The circle is then repeated with another partner. If there are six males in the house and six females, six complete circles are attempted.

It is most important that nothing interrupt the circles. A telephone call, a look at a newspaper, a TV commercial, leaving the premises, mean that the circle should be stopped at that point. This is a concentrated effort to gain total satiation and to be totally drained sexually so that Nirvana can be entered.

In this state at the end of the agreed number of cycles, all gather in the exercise room for the great meditational release. Everyone does lotus meditation, where everyone opens to see what will come through. In this state some of the practitioners go into Nirvana and experience ultimate bliss.

The time from the maximum completions of the Kundalini Cycle to the beginning of the sexual fast is a time of sadness and letting down. The yogi and the yogin meet each other for a sexual opportunity twice a day. We find that right after kundalini, sex is still turned from an opportunity into a copulation; after a couple of days the pace slackens and there are some days toward the beginning of the fast when no copulation occurs. It is totally up to the people involved. There is no requirement to do anything except meet and snuggle.

PERFECTION

It may take months for the sexual performance of many house members to settle into the rhythm of the house. It should be noted that only the dyadic couple know what occurs within the privacy of the sleeping quarters for the ritual copulations. If either partner cares only for his or her own pleasure and is exploitive, not selfless, this fact is brought up at the general house meeting; but if either partner's drive is simply too low, it is not discussed unless he or she cannot make at least the single orgasm each day. The body adjusts in the regularity of orgasms; it becomes more matter-of-fact as time progresses. You might think that with having sex so often the need diminishes, but that's not the way it works. Miss a day and you'll really be hard up!

It may be that in your house you will never reach the perfection of a complete moon cycle. The members may be too old to gain the rhythm, or the necessary stimulation may be lacking.

Do not try for artificial stimulation. The mind must be taught to control the body. If all else fails, simple increase the frequency of partner exchange.

OTHER SEXUAL CONTACTS

Because the house is quite open and behaves very naturally with a lot of loving, touching, and contact, there will often be occasions when couples make love at times other than those required by ritual. This is as it should be; for anyone can make love to anyone, and a group of people can make love as a group if they desire. Two males or two females may also without blame enjoy sharing an encounter with each other. It is most important, though, that for the health of the house all the bathing and purification steps be taken before such encounters and that household duties and work are completed on schedule. One type of behavior is totally unacceptable—that is teasing and undue coyness. It is altogether unfair for one person to lead another into expecting a sexual encounter with an orgasmic release unless he or she intends to fulfill the promise. In the outside world the term "tease" has come to be used for people who exhibit behavior of this type. It should be avoided. Don't start a tease situation which you do not expect to follow through to completion. The converse is also true—don't push yourself on an unwilling partner. By whatever name, this is rape, and is totally taboo. Whereas a little teasing might occasionally be permissible just in fun, rape is not allowed under any circumstances.

A DAY IN A TANTRIC HOUSE

Ideally the people of a Tantric house work for the house and do not have to go out and punch the time clocks of modern commerce; though here again we are dealing with an idealized situation. When the time clock has to be used, the schedule within the house must be adapted to accommodate the people who are punching the clock.

From the sounding of the wakeup signal to the greeting of the sun, a silent period is observed in the house. The waking-buzzer is set for approximately one half hour before sunrise. The members go to the bathing area; after evacuating their bowels they go through the purification procedures described in chapter 5. Each dyadic couple works together to make sure that all steps are completed. They spend eight minutes together in the bath; they go through the cool shower together. They dry off and go to the exercise room. A few minutes of quiet cuddling and petting are allowed while all wait for the rim of the sun to come over the horizon. (On cloudy days, of course, the ritual is started when the second hand of the clock gets to the specific time defined by the almanac.) At the appropriate time, the complete Welcoming The Sun ritual is performed, including pelvic tilt exercises with yoni contraction and lingam expansion.

A nesting of eight minutes follows the sun greeting. This is a quiet period where no other motion or action is permitted. After the quiet period the couples may do as they wish, except those responsible for cooking, who must have breakfast on the table 32 minutes after the close of the sun-greeting ritual.

After breakfast, washing, grooming, and dressing, the members go to work, taking lunch with them. They return about 6 P.M. At this time they take off work clothes and proceed directly to the exercise room where they go through 32 minutes of muscle-relaxing and mind-releasing exercises. After this period, they go to the bathing area and do evening purifications. When these are complete, the cooks again have approximately 32 minutes to get the evening meal on the table. During this interval another silent time is observed. After the evening meal has been enjoyed, there are usually several hours of discretionary time when members can do as they wish. This ends with the final visit to the bathroom before the evening's first ritual copulation.

Houses may rearrange schedules to fit their needs. The only thing to remember is that cleanliness before any sexual contact is of paramount importance in the Tantric way. Exterior genitalia and the interior of the lingam are cleansed before sexual contact is made. This may seem a minor point, but a little thought shows how practical a requirement it is; and once the habit is established, since it signals future sexual pleasure it does not detract from lovemaking.

Any time too rigid a schedule is established in a house and somebody in the house starts to say such things as, "The book requires that we do this," the thinking of the house should be reevaluated. A Tantric house is a relaxed, pleasant place to live. Although the continuation of the monthly and yearly cycles is important in Tantric life, they should not be made into a rod to beat members into submission. Laughter, water play, harmless comments and silly, perhaps childish games of charades, forfeits, truth or consequences, will lighten the atmosphere. Happiness must be the order of the house, not drudgery and absolute obedience to the arbitrary dictates of some other human being. If the schedule does not fit your house, make a new one! Make it happier. Change couples at different rates. Gather together in the exercise room more often—or less often. Do not change for the sake of change. Once you have established a procedure, try at least to keep it together for several months, because it is in the non-changing but ever-changing ritual that Tantrists find themselves.

HETEROSEXUALITY AND HOMOSEXUALITY

In today's world, most members of Tantric houses might be described as partially bisexual. In work and in play some homosexual contact is almost inevitable. It is often found that a male knows how to rouse a male, knows what he wants, more than a female does; and it is certainly true that the female may know what the female wants far more explicitly than does a male. By not avoiding homosexual contacts, by not being uptight about them, heterosexuals can learn many secrets which enable them to bring even more pleasure to future partners. It sometimes takes males a long time to adjust to the idea of being caressed by another male. There is plenty of time, and gradually with love and understanding on both sides, the barriers begin to fall away. It is inevitably true that when two males have shared a sexual experience they become less threatened by one another and more tolerant of the roster system of the house.

THE GREAT YEAR CYCLE

Tantra relies on the two interlocking cycles of the heavens. First is the moon, second is the sun, and additional ritual observances are appropriate for the moon's waxing and waning. The sun tends to be considered as male; yet in conjunction with Mother Earth, the sun produces fertility, so in its fertility aspect it is female.

The year is marked off into segments by great sun festivals. The sun moves relatively slowly in the ever-changing skies, so slavish adherence to the exact date of an equinox or a solstice is not required. For example, in 1987 the longest day at 50 degrees North was 16 hours 44 minutes. A week earlier, it was 16 hours 40 minutes; a week later it was 16 hours 42 minutes. So unless the house is heavily into astrology, moving the solstice celebration should cause little concern.

Starting at the fall equinox as winter approaches, the sun is heavily male-aspected. This is the hunting season. Some houses make a deliberate foray and hunt a deer. They always try to kill an old buck. The house likes to skin out its own deer and store the meat; for in this way members reconnect themselves to the old natural ways. This ritual slaying of the deer must nowadays wait for the opening of the local hunting season. At the full moon following that date, the spirit of the slain deer is contacted in meditation; it is told that it can now progress through the next cycle of reincarnation and that it has been released so it can go to an incarnation at a higher level. Ideally this special lotus meditation and communication occur after the full-moon Kundalini Circle ceremony. After the hunt, an additional circle ceremony is often done purely for the propitiation of the dead animal's spirit to make sure it has in fact progressed. If it is inappropriate for your house to kill a deer, another animal can be substituted.

The next great sun festival occurs at winter solstice. Throughout this longest night of the year, house members give gifts to each other and visit. They stay up all night waiting to make absolutely sure that the sun will reappear the next morning. Wines are drunk in remembrance of the warmth of the sun that generated the vintage. Oranges and other golden fruits are eaten. During this night, five different meals are eaten; often they include beans and rice. The meals are intended to show that prosperity has been in the house for the year and will come back to the house more abundantly in the following year; that is why swelling foods like beans and rice are used. A swelling dessert is also eaten, perhaps English Christmas pudding or "spotted dick," which contains many raisins in the dough.

If there is another Tantric house in the neighborhood, the senior couple from each house exchange houses for the night. They come to the house bringing gifts, often firewood and bread. The firewood and bread are kept for the whole year and are replaced only when new wood and bread are brought in the following year. Sometimes the senior couple will only go outside, circle the house three times sunwise (clockwise), and reenter, pretending to be strangers bringing wood and bread.

At spring equinox the female-aspected fertility sun is welcomed back. This is the beginning of the fertility season and usually some quick-growing seeds are planted. Many of the females will be large with child if they conceived at the great summer solstice fertility festival. This is the happiest time of the whole year; things are beginning to sprout and grow, babies are coming into the world, and warmth and sunlight are returning.

Many houses perform a great sun-greeting festival where all who are able participate one with another in doing a sun greeting for this one morning.

SUMMER SOLSTICE IS SPECIAL

Conception at summer solstice results in births at the spring equinox. This is very nice in a Tantric house, for the majority of the females who want to bear children have them at the same time. All the diaper stages, all the midnight feedings, all the equipment become a shared responsibility which everyone

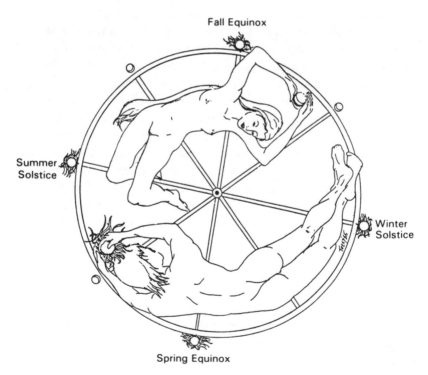

Figure 18.   The year cycle.

understands. Interestingly enough, babies born in late March tend to have a higher IQ than those born at other times of the year. This may simply be because of the way the public school system is arranged in northern countries; we do not know. In winter and spring, pregnancy is more comfortable than one that comes to term in the heat of summer. Summer solstice is thus the fertility festival of all fertility festivals, and the females are encouraged to conceive on this night of nights—if they wish to. Of course, the choice is their own.

Just as at the winter solstice, members of the house do not normally sleep during this night. This is the night when members try to find out how long the ritual Kundalini Circles can be sustained. In younger houses the circles can be maintained all night. Perhaps surprisingly, in some of the older houses most of the night can be taken up with the circles, although some fail after the eighth or ninth ritual copulation.

This series of ritual orgasms allows the female to select any partner she chooses to father her child. It takes only the private insertion or removal of the diaphragm for fertilization to occur with the partner she wishes. It is best if she arranges that her first partner of the night be the one she selects.

Somehow the maypole got displaced in Europe but is retained in India at midsummer. Tantric houses bring in a pole and dance around it for their midsummer festival.

This brings the year cycle fully around. It is pictorially summarized in figure 18. It can take great ingenuity to make the cycles and circles fit one within another. The lunar month menstrual cycle is the least subject to change, whereas the sun cycle progresses more slowly; so in reconciling cycles, it is better to move the equinox and solstice rites than to change the lunar cycle.

THE WEEK CYCLE

Many people try to fit a secondary week cycle into the moon cycle of 29½ days. This is a difficult job and one which a house should try to avoid. Unfortunately we all suffer from it. If you work a standard week in the mundane world, the energies often peak on Sunday and are lowest on Thursday. Do your best to fit the moon cycle observances into the week in such a way that the full moon observances occur on a Sunday and the new moon ones on a Thursday. Some houses find they must arrange both new moon and full moon festivals to fall on either a Saturday or a Sunday because the festival simply cannot be squeezed into a normal work day.

THE MONTH CYCLE

There are many ways of looking at the cycle of a Tantric month. A psychiatrist might say the oral satisfaction of food is exchanged for the genital satisfaction of sex and loving; thus balance is maintained. An older person sees that mental activity replaces physical activity and balance is maintained. A physician might see it as a way of exercising all the functions of the body—physical, mental, sexual, and emotional. The Tantrist sees it as a training program. Knowing what is to be makes today's experiences worthwhile and meaningful. Sexual pressure is felt by people who do not live within the cycle, and this means they never learn to control their passion so that it can be given free rein at the appropriate time.

THE EIGHTFOLD PATH

Because the seven chakras and Beyond constitute the mystical sacred eight, eights are included in all ritual timing and numerology. The cycle within the month is also an eightfold path, as shown in figure 17 on page 123. The segments appear to be of varying lengths; however, any Tantrist will tell you a moment of bliss is equivalent to hours of mundane living, so in fact the cycles are of more equal length than is evident.

PART
THREE

ACTIVATING AND ILLUMINATING THE CHAKRAS

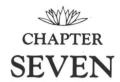

CHAPTER
SEVEN

The Chakras

DESPITE THE WESTERN urge to define and clarify, the chakras are indefinable. They are psychic realities which exist in your own reality construct. What I experience when I enter a chakra is similar to what you experience, but it is not identical. The colors, symbols (sigils), gods, goddesses, sounds, smells, textures, and all the other descriptions are only signposts to the chakras; they are not the chakra itself. Comprehension of the chakras is gained only through your own sudden empirical insight—the "aha!" experience—in, for, and of yourself.

The ancient Hindu writings that explain spiritual truths seem confused in their descriptions of the chakras. The confusion is brought about by a lack of understanding of the concept and a lack of subjective thinking. The ancient scriptures are in fact one. When one writer compares a chakra to a berserk elephant, and another to the sound of hard drum beats, and yet another to the feeling of evacuating the bowels, they are all actually describing the same indescribable chakra as they best perceive it in their reality at a particular moment in time. This depends on the percentage of each mode of awareness they are using and on their emotional feelings at the time of writing the description. Tomorrow they might describe it differently. Table 2 on page 44 is an attempt to put together the descriptions given by several writers who obviously had differing percentages of their -voyant, -audient, -olfactory, etc., selves working while they were writing.

If you read one of the thousands of textbooks presently available describing the chakras, you will find differing precise and exact descriptions. We believe that this is at best the writer's own feeling for the chakra he or she is describing. At worst it is only the repetition of someone else's work—which may or may not be based on the old writings or on personal experience. Recent efforts to replace the gods and goddesses in the chakra with a single "Jesus force" show complete lack of understanding of the chakra concept.

What follows is our best effort to describe our perception of the chakras using both the terminology of the old writings, where it can be understood, and modern Western language. Read with understanding, and do not reject new ideas until you have the same awareness as the guru.

LOCATION OF THE CHAKRAS

We have heard hundreds of people allege that a chakra is located at a specific place in the body. It is very difficult for most untrained psychics to comprehend the meaning of a chakra, so they simply place it at a specific location, revealing their stupidity and lack of comprehension. What they are trying to do is make objective something which is altogether subjective. They are trying to tidy it up, put it into a pretty box, and tie it with the strong cord of Western linear thinking.

Think for a moment of "I" and "Me." You have a mind. You might say, "It is in my brain." If you are a little more aware, you will say, "It is in my brain, in my spinal column, and distributed throughout my body in the form of nerve fibers." But still you have a location; "my mind" can be conceived of as being mainly in the head with small pieces that you can imagine distributed elsewhere. But where is "I"? We know that people with large portions of their brain destroyed still carry on living. "I" is still present somewhere.

A simplistic representation is that "I" is an etheric body which is the twin of "Me's" body and occupies the same space as "Me" except when "I" leaves in such exercises as astral travel. If you imagine now that the etheric body does not necessarily have the same shape as "Me's" body, and if you now realize that awareness is retained in the "I," not in the "Me," then you are well along the road to understanding where the chakras are.

For a moment, imagine that you are viewing an etheric body which actually has the exact shape of a standard human body. You can now say that the base chakra is located some-where near the posterior yoni and in fact is between this and the genitalia. It might appear to you as a small horizontal disk threaded on the etheric representation of the spinal column; and to it and through it flow all the etheric nerves (ethers) that control the action of the posterior yoni, the feet, and the legs.

Any time we discuss the location of a chakra, we mean its location in its etheric body – which may or may not correspond to a location in the mundane body. When the two occupy the same space, the locations coincide; but since the two are not attached to each other in any physical way, they do not neces-sarily continue to coincide from moment to moment.

THE IDA AND THE PINGALA

You have a spine. It is assumed that when the etheric and the mundane bodies occupy the same space, two channels carry sub-tle information from the base of the spine to the brain. These are the Ida (which starts on the left side of the base) and the Pingala (which starts on the right side). See figure 19 on page 142. These two spiral upward around the spine and join together at the brow. The etheric counterpart of the spine is a very fine channel called the Chitrini. When the two bodies are superimposed, this would run up the center of the spine. Each chakra is considered

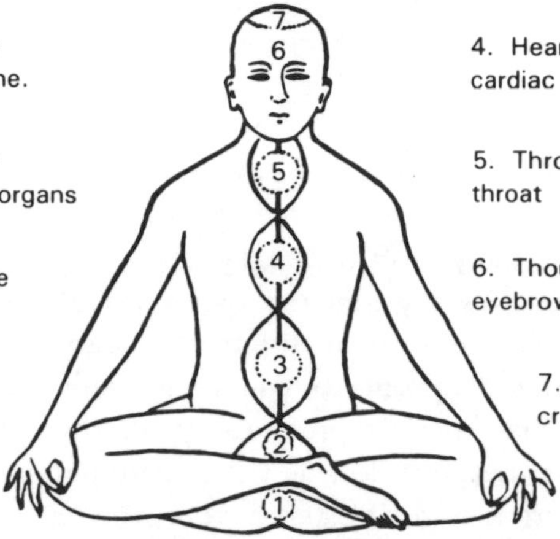

The Seven Principal Chakras

1. Base: at the
base of the spine.

2. Pelvic: over
the generative organs

3. Navel: at the
solar plexus

4. Heart: at the
cardiac plexus

5. Throat: in the
throat

6. Thought: between the
eyebrows

7. Crown: at the
crown of the head

Figure 19. Ida and pingala. The intertwining lines represent the
direction of the positive (pingala) and negative (ida) forces of prana.
The central channel is chitrini.

to be a wheel of light no bigger than the physical spine, which is
threaded on the Chitrini and held in place by the Ida and the
Pingala.

Each chakra can be thought of as a controlling section for
part of the mind which is resident in that part of the body. Just
as "I" controls the mind which controls the whole body, so the
chakra controls the etheric impulses for the nerves that are
"near" it physically. It is the mind of the body that is near.
Although we know that the mind controls the nerves which
twitch the foot by communicating down the nerves of the spinal
column to the nerves in the foot, still the chakra ultimately
controls all the nerves in its sphere of influence and all the
feelings associated with them, just as "I" should control "Me." In
other words, just as the mind is diffused throughout the body,
so is the "I."

DESCRIPTION OF THE CHAKRAS

In the meditation section, you learned that all things have at least six modes of being comprehended. In stem meditation you learned to concentrate on an object with all these modes of understanding. It is with the same modes that you will attempt to comprehend a chakra. Do not take anybody's clumsy description of a chakra literally. The words used to describe it are words meaningful to the person doing the description. Even to that person the words change from minute to minute.

A good example is in the color blue. Blue is symbolic of a relatively "up" person and aura: the light blue sky; yet if I am out on the street and I see a terrible accident involving people wearing blue, for a little while after that time the color blue will be negative for me. Thus if I am trying to think of a chakra that has the color blue, I have to put away thoughts of the accident and think instead of the meaning to me of the chakra itself, not of the color blue. Blue is meant as a mind-trigger that will make your mind comprehend a certain feeling. If I use the term "angry red," probably a dirty dusty red will come to your mind and when you think of that specific color of red you can feel anger. You can also feel anger when you remember that last fight you had with the garage mechanic or your annoyance at the sound of a mosquito in the night or the anger at that bounced check or at the rotten smell of garbage not taken out. Let us look at what type of memory the various anger-triggers may be to you. Table 5 on page 144 may help you categorize them. You have in your head a thousand different impressions that when recalled may put you into anger. The body itself responds with flows of adrenaline and gets itself prepared to fight—but can you describe anger? Can you describe joy? Or happiness? Or love?

Everyone's descriptions would be different. Because the chakras are psychic constructs, they are difficult to describe in mundane words and have often been said to be "beyond thought." Perhaps they could be likened to magnetism, which is

Table 5. Experiences and Associations

Experience	Type of Association	Type of Awareness
Angry Red	Color	Voyant
Mosquito	Sound	Audient
Bounced Check	Symbol	Voyant
Garage Mechanic	Emotional	Sentient
Garbage	Smell	Olfactory

in iron but is *not* the actual iron. They are, as the old books say: That, not This, yet they are in fact *in* This.

When you first use our signposts and keys to understand the chakras, you must transcend the thought of the chakras and use petal meditation to go beyond your mind into the psychic chakra. Eventually, after doing both stem and petal meditation on a given chakra for several hours, you will have that "aha!" experience. Suddenly you will totally comprehend in your own awareness what this specific chakra is! Even when you have had the "aha!" experience, you will still find it difficult to describe to someone else. It is not easy to quantify an idea.

THE ILLUMINATION AND ACTIVATION OF THE CHAKRAS

Each chakra can be approached either from below during ascent, or from above during descent. During ascent, the chakras are activated by the respective goddesses resident in them. They are illuminated by the god-presence during descent when you bring illumination back from beyond the thousand-petaled lotus. Thus each chakra has symbology associated with its two states: the activated state as you move upward, and the illuminated state as you descend. During ascent each chakra is entered in turn; you experience and transcend the emotions; then the goddess moves you on to the next set of experiences to be transcended. You must actually experience the emotions with every fiber of your being before you can transcend them. During descent, order and balance are brought with the inspiration from the transcendent illumination that your journey beyond the lotus gave you.

If you look again at Table 2 on page 44 you will see how this fits together with the phases of the moon. You climb up the chakras as the moon waxes. Then, having been close to Nirvana, you bring illumination back down with you as you return with the waning moon. This is shown diagrammatically in figure 20a.

Each time you complete the cycle, you bring a little more illumination back down with you and you start upward again with more understanding. This can be represented by the spiral of development shown in figure 20b where the shattered crystal represents entering into the thousand-petaled lotus.

"Up" and "down" are physical representations of growth that occurs with time. We have no adequate description of the journey except "up" and "down." The spiral starts at a point (Self), expands you outward and upward, and then brings you down and out to the world with new understanding.

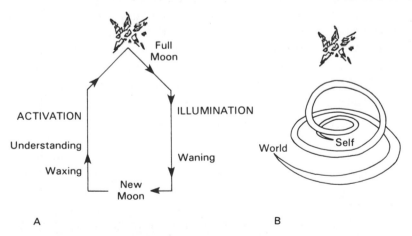

Figure 20. Illumination of the chakras. (A) Ascending and descending and (B) spiral of development.

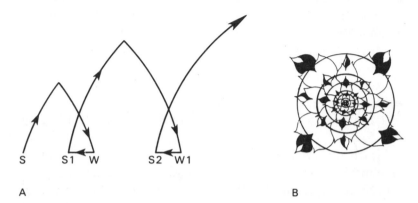

Figure 21.   The spiral and the lotus.

After a few trips around the spiral you will leave it and enter full Nirvana-consciousness. As you work more and more at traveling up and returning with illumination, you will gain more enlightenment. Figure 21a is one way of representing your journey through time and awareness. Starting at the center, where the S stands for Self, you proceed up through the chakras on your spiral of increase. Then with illumination you return downward to the world at point W on the spiral. You live in the world a little while and your flame of illumination grows dim. Then you start another progress represented by S1. This takes you higher and further. Now as you descend you bring more illumination with you, until you return to your world at W1.

After several months of training, your start and finish points grow very close together and your progression takes on the appearance of a spiral contained in a cylinder. The infinite height of the cylinder represents the Nirvanic state. It is no coincidence that the representation is that of the overlaid petals of a lotus figure 21b.

The three-dimensional spiral is our attempt to represent a multi-dimensional concept which is in fact spiraling through time and space.

On a two-dimensional plane, each trip around the spiral reduces itself to a circle. As we move around the Circle of Life, we spend seven years in each quadrant. In the first seven years, we gain control of our limbs and our bowels. The second seven years bring us to full reproductive maturity. In the third seven years we start to learn to control our sexual drives. We become craftsmen in the way in which we gain fulfillment. In the fourth seven years we fall in love, marry, and start raising a family. Thus to complete one turn around the circle takes 28 years.

The next segment, age 28 to 35, takes us to a point where we are gaining much new knowledge and learning to control our place in the world; thus it is very similar to the first seven years. It has the same type of attributes. For males, the mother is

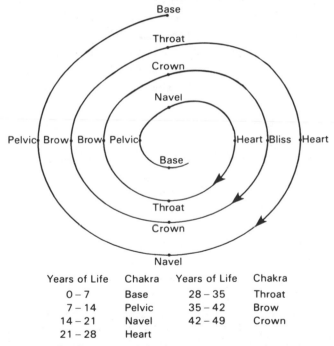

Years of Life	Chakra	Years of Life	Chakra
0 – 7	Base	28 – 35	Throat
7 – 14	Pelvic	35 – 42	Brow
14 – 21	Navel	42 – 49	Crown
21 – 28	Heart		

Figure 22.   Stations on the circle of life. Bliss is ruled by the heart. The base then becomes illuminated and uplifted. The crown can be uplifted and then brought down.

replaced by the wife and the guru; for women the mother is replaced by the husband and the guru. It is a slightly higher level of the first seven years. Thus we are on an upward spiral. Each of these Stations of Life (as they are called) correlates with one of the chakras. We progress upward to the Crown in our 49th year. Then we begin to return back down the spiral into our retirement, repeating childish things and eventually returning to the base, where we will become one with the earth from which we were formed. This is shown in figure 22.

Since we rise up through the chakras and return down through them, the spiral repeats itself. There are seven chakras on the journey through life and seven chakras in retirement—a total of fourteen chakras to be mastered. We dwell in each for seven years for a total life span of 98 years—a little more than most expect. Since there are four stations on each turn of the spiral, we have a total of $3^{1}/_{2}$ turns. This total of $3^{1}/_{2}$ turns is represented in Tantra by the $3^{1}/_{2}$ turns that the serpent Kundalini is coiled sleeping in you just below the base chakra. Many interpretations are possible for the $3^{1}/_{2}$ turns, but the explanation above seems to us to form a natural Thatness.

GODS AND GODDESSES IN THE CHAKRAS

Each chakra contains a resident god and goddess. It is important to understand they are all aspects of Shiva and Shakti and, further, that the picture of the God-ess is meant only as an earthplane representation of something which is beyond thought. The picture of the multi-armed Shiva is a finite anthropomorphic representation of a god, but the essence of Shiva is beyond our common picture. It might be said to represent god's will or purpose, or god's reality. These are ideomorphic representations of the god—ideas you might have about the god or about what it represents. But Shiva is beyond this representation, just as he is beyond anthropomorphic representation. In desperation you might say, "Well, Shiva represents the force of god's will," or "The light of the god in the universe." The guru would respond, "Those ideas are mineromorphic." For again they are representations of the god in terms that you might use to talk about the force of gravity or the force of the wind. They are terms associated with the mundane plane in which we live—and Shiva is beyond this concept. So when we tell you that Shiva in this aspect is a red god covered with gray ash, that representation is not to be taken literally, for the essence of Shiva in this aspect is beyond that representation. The picture is given as a mind key that will lock you into thoughts of Shiva that are totally beyond mundane words.

The picture is to be transcended. The guru says, "The understanding of a chakra begins with a simple verbal pictogram."

TYPES OF CHAKRAS

Tantrists recognize seven chakras (see figure 19, page 142) divided into three groups.

Group 1) The five chakras of the mundane;

Group 2) The chakra of thought;

Group 3) The chakra Beyond.

Sometimes an eighth chakra is mentioned, called the Red-Jeweled Chakra. It seems, though, that this one was added purely for the benefit of teachers, and modern Tantrists rarely use it. It is the chakra of the Red Lotus of Eight Petals, which is said to lie just below the heart chakra. It is described as an island of gems, inside which is an altar where the student must worship his or her teacher by adding a gem to the gems already in the chakra. The new gem can be either a mundane ruby (for those who are wealthy and have little understanding) or a gem of knowledge (for those who are poor and have much understanding). It is the chakra of devotional meditation on your guru. When you meditate on this chakra you give the guru more knowledge, more wisdom, and better health.

The Mundane Chakras

The five mundane or operational chakras control the entire body except the mind. These five chakras are named after their height location on the Chitrini in the etheric body:

1) Base—at the base of the sexual organ and the anus;

2) Pelvic—at the top of the sexual organ and below the navel;[1]

3) Navel—in the region of the navel;

4) Heart—in the region of the heart;

5) Throat—at the lower end of the throat.[2]

They are also the chakras of the senses:

1) sight

2) hearing

3) taste

4) smell

5) touch

They are associated with the five organs of the senses:

1) eyes

2) ears

---

[1]Called "pelvic" so that no one will be offended by calling it the "genital" chakra.

[2]The throat chakra controls the mundane aspects of the head.

3) tongue

4) nose

5) skin

They are also associated with the five mundane "airs":

1) the breeze of the eyelids

2) belching and farting

3) sneezing

4) yawning

5) nourishment-through-air[3]

and with the five vital airs:

1) prana (the breath of life)

2) apana (expelling air—controlling wind, excrement, urine, semen)

3) samana (fire of the body—nourishment)

4) udana (exhalation)

5) vyana (digestion)

and with the five observances:

1) cleanliness

2) contentment

3) self-perfection (body and senses)

4) self-analysis

5) attentiveness

---

[3]When breathed in the Ha-tha manner, air gives the body vital nourishment.

and with the five restraints:

1) no injury of others

2) truthfulness

3) no theft

4) spiritual conduct

5) no greed

The Chakra of Thought

This is the brow chakra, the chakra of the mind. In its great subtlety, it is entirely different from the five which precede it. The two etheric channels (Ida and Pingala) join the Chitrini at this point, and the whole consciousness proceeds onward. Here the main part of "I" resides. It is located in the etheric body in the location of the "third eye" and when the two bodies are together, it can sometimes be contacted through the third eye.

In some ways it may be thought of as "I" and as a coordinator and controller of all the mundane chakras, unifying their five-foldedness. Through this control "I" reigns supreme, having understood and appreciated all the pleasures and experiences the five-fold chakras bring to "Me." All is brought together in this chakra.

This melding of all—both satiation and fasting, both material and spiritual—results in something which is much more than its individual parts. Transcendence of this chakra leads to the thousand-petaled lotus of the secret chakra.

The Crown or Secret Chakra

Whatever name anyone calls the thousand-petaled chakra, whatever description is given it, all are correct; for it contains all within itself, and it is contained within everything. To describe it to the uninitiated is futile. To describe it to the initiated will surely start an argument, for comprehension of this chakra is beyond intuition. At its center is the void, the Ultimate, which is "served in secret by all the devas." It is an experience beyond the mind, just as the brow chakra is an experience beyond the mundane. Through it we find illumination and Nirvana. Imagine a ball resting on a plane. This might represent the mundane. Now imagine a "something" resting on a sphere having the same relation to the sphere as the ball had to the plane. This might represent the brow. Now imagine "X" in relation to "something." This may give you a little comprehension of the secret chakra.

Throughout the following descriptions you are encouraged to spend a great deal of time—three or four days—with at least two hours meditation a day in learning each chakra in turn. Each meditation must be done at the correct phase of the moon.

SIGNPOSTS THAT WILL GET YOU INTO THE CHAKRA

It is up to you to understand each signpost in as many modes of your own awareness as you can bring to it. For example, you must ideally understand it as a taste, a texture, a sound, an emotional feeling, a symbol, and a smell. Since there are signposts for each of the six modes of comprehension, plus a god or a goddess, an animal, an element, and a material, it is difficult initially to apply six modes of comprehension to all of these eleven signposts. We recommend that you start by comprehending each signpost at the following three levels:

• the meaning;

• the idea behind the meaning;

• the spiritual truth behind the idea behind the meaning.

If you can comprehend each of the eleven signposts we will give you for each chakra in this way, you will approach understanding. Remember that ultimately your understanding is something you must gain intuitively through an "aha!" experience. Once you have gained that understanding, you will be able to enter the chakra as soon as you think of it.

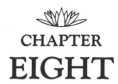

CHAPTER
EIGHT

Ascending Kundalini: Activating the Chakras

EVERY DAY OF a Tantrist's life is different because each day's spiritual exercises are based on the moon cycle. The moon cycle interacts with the days of the week and the seasons of the year in an extremely complex round; so in the lifetime of any Tantrist on this plane of existence, the conditions for the work will never exactly replicate themselves.

Each month, every sincere Tantrist attempts to complete the cycle shown in figure 17 on page 123. In this chapter the guru will examine the time from new moon to full moon: the ascending, growing, activating phase. The descending phase is examined in chapter 9. These ascents and descents are keyed to your own body and to the chakras in general. You are allowed two days to master each ascending step and its chakra.

The guru recommends these steps.

1) Do a stem meditation (page 72) using the suggested signposts and illustrations. Get inside yourself and the chakra, and comprehend its metaphorical meaning. Each month you will gain new understanding of your own nature, the nature of the world, and the meaning of the chakra. Up to one hour a day may be spent in this stem work.

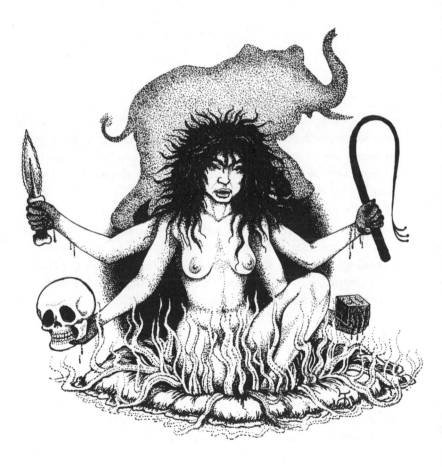

Figure 23.   Dakini.

2) When the stem meditation is complete, do the ritual with the group, making changes as the group's consciousness and understanding improve.

3) When the ritual is complete, do a fifteen-minute petal meditation (page 80) with appropriate safeguards to see what guidance you can receive, both individually and as a group. Then it is usual to come down by taking a cool drink and being close with your partner(s). Some like quiet music, others massage. Whatever your preference, this should be a gentle and soothing reentry into the world. When everyone is reintegrated with their bodies, a discussion of results is in order. It is not unusual for several members of a group to find they have received the same guidance. You should act on the guidance; otherwise it will cease.

The approach to each chakra must be done at the correct phase of the moon, after the correct dietary and sexual work has been completed. If you simply read this material without doing the meditations and ritual work associated with it, you will gain scant understanding from your guru; but the decision is yours.

ACTIVATING THE BASE CHAKRA

The base chakra represents raw, basic, uncontrolled instincts. It is the underlying, undisciplined frenzy of nature. It might be thought of as the goddess Kali in her most rampant savage modes. In Tantra it is represented by the goddess Dakini, who has four red hands. She has a whip, and her hands are dipped in blood (see figure 23). If you cast your mind back to the time when nature was struggling to establish itself as a living force rising from the primeval swamp, you get some feel for the raw rugged energy of this chakra. You cannot get more primitive than this. We will now discuss the signposts for activating the base chakra.

Symbol: The symbol is a cube. It is very hard, and is sharply defined. If you look closely at the cube, you will see it is like some obscene jigsaw puzzle, made up of millions of particles all of different shapes. The closer you look, the more you marvel that this indescribable variety of shapes can be brought together and controlled in the framework of a cube. It represents all the diverse forces of nature being firmly controlled by the powerful goddess Dakini.

Color: The color is a nasty greenish-yellow. You can compare it to the color of violent diarrhea. It is not a blended, continuous color, but one made up of all the various pieces of nasty fecal matter you have ever seen.

Emotion: Here is the sullen, resentful anger of someone who is at the mercy of forces way beyond his control, who is being tossed and flung in the middle of a hurricane or an earthquake, or is being held against his will as the lava from a volcano approaches. Tinged into this sullen resentful anger there is envy of the power of the person(s) controlling him. The anger explodes into futile frenzy. You throw yourself against the forces and in doing so are completely frustrated.

Element: Earth which is just about to be formed from the primeval soup of the world in the turmoil of creation. The earth is swamp-like, oozing, and very dangerous. One false step and you will fall into the muck and mire.

Sound: A frenzy of deep, dark heavy drums. There is no rhythm. It is a jumble of sound that cannot be understood by your mind.

The mantra is LA$\underline{M}$,[1] the broken LA-$\underline{M}$, not a continuous sound as you have been accustomed to hearing in Hindu mantras. The silent $\underline{M}$ is the bodily hum vibrating at such a deep note that it affects the upper legs and the anus.

---

[1] Throughout the text, we will use $\underline{M}$ underlined to signify the hum with closed mouth after a mantric chant.

Animal: A berserk elephant. The elephant with all its power is running amok. It turns and kills its keeper. It shakes its head in fury. It charges through a house and destroys it. It has no direction. It is out of control.

Material: Sulphur, boiling and churning in a vat. In its depth you can see raw red heat. One tiny drop of boiling sulphur touches your anus. The pain and comprehension begin to bring you into the material of this chakra.

Texture: The texture is that of slimy, greasy, greenish-yellow mucus. You know how awful it feels.

Smell: This is the worst possible stench you can imagine. Whatever you have smelled that is totally awful, that is the smell of this chakra. It combines every repulsive smell you can imagine.

Taste: The taste is very easily imagined. It is that of a raw rotten egg yolk. The egg yolk stinks, and the stink is transferred into your mouth and throat.

Goddess: The goddess of this chakra is Dakini, the ultimate, underlying nature goddess. She is all-powerful, yet, to be fully in control, she needs Shiva. She is angry that she needs him. She does not understand why she needs him and she is frantic that he is not yet there. She is trying to bring all her primeval emotions into control and she is gradually succeeding. She already controls the baser elements of the earth; but she is in a frenzy to control her own emotions.

In succeeding chakras the following instruction is omitted because it is essentially the same, though with changed signposts for each in turn.

Spend up to one hour sitting quietly in stem meditation thinking on these eleven facets of the base chakra, and push all these feelings *down* into the anus. As you think of them, try to think what it would be like coming up through the anus and into the base chakra; for the anus is the gateway that gets you into it. When you can comprehend these primeval forces, the fact that they are very necessary and that you have to go through shit to comprehend them will help you learn the meaning of the chakra.

Ritual for Activating the
Base Chakra

This is the ritual that gets Tantrists into a lot of trouble with the establishment, especially when the ritual is carried beyond conventionally accepted levels of behavior. It occurs after the time of heavy brutal work and toward the end of the sexual fast. The people of the house have been doing manual labor, and have been fasting sexually. They may be bruised; they may have blisters and abrasions. Preferably, they have all been doing work that makes them sweat, and of a nature they don't like. If someone doesn't like cleaning the toilet or the cellar, that's the job to be done. An apocryphal story told about Mohandas Gandhi relates that when his wife resisted cleaning the toilets, he told her she had to do it just as everyone else did — and especially she must if she thought she was above it, because obviously her protest meant that she had not transcended the base chakra.

A small fire is kindled in the exercise room. On it is placed an iron pot of sulphur. The yogins cut whippy, flexible sticks. (In northern lands the favorite tree for this is birch; in India, Tantrists occasionally use whips made from the hide of a specially sacrificed cow.)

No purifying bath or washing is done before this ritual. Yogis and yogins come in stinking from the mire, wearing a sash of obscene yellow fabric around their waist; its end hangs down behind like a tail. They rub on their skin any handy dirt or mud, and can liberally smear the buttocks and pelvis with grime.

They come into the room stamping in a broken pattern. The yogins slap or hit the yogis with their sticks or simply buffet them with their behinds. The yogis are allowed only to defend themselves. If the group is incapable of hitting each other with some sort of control, it is best to hit yourself; but there must be real, significant pain. Where a single Tantrist works alone, self-flagellation is employed. In many groups pummeling with fists is allowed and bruising is encouraged. This may be necessary at the first group ritual, but it is certainly not necessary in subsequent group rituals.

The members form groups of four each: males with males, females with females. One member of the small group stands passively while the other three join hands to form a small circle around him or her. They use their bodies to buffet him or her from one to the next. He or she must not resist. After about four minutes of this treatment, another person replaces "It" to take a turn as the passive, buffeted one while the former "It" gets the feeling of power and control.

When everyone has been buffeted, the whole group comes together and falls on one another in a writhing frenzy of conflict. This is primordial frenzy. Any part below the waist can be slapped or grabbed and twisted. The lingam and yoni are off limits, but testicles are not. They can be squeezed until the man submits.

A special note on the anterior yoni: Some groups have encouraged the penetration of the anterior yoni with fingers or lingam during this frenzied exchange. The posterior yoni is the gateway and it is to be opened in some way during the ritual. It is recommended that rubber gloves be available to the participants for this exchange if the house members consider it a requirement.

Getting into this ritual is even more important for the nice, clean members of the house than for the more earthy members. They must be able to transcend the primordial passions and control them, and this ritual is the means of gaining that experience.

Guided Meditation

When the ritual is complete and everyone is exhausted from the effort, a guided meditation is done. Words such as the following will help to guide the house members into the base chakra:

Come with me now, and I will take you back in time. See
your ancestors. They are hairy, naked creatures living in caves.
They are eating raw meat. Go back now further. There are
dinosaurs. You are living in a fetid jungle. The swamps bubble
and smell. The sky is dull orange. Smoke and decay are everywhere. You move further back. You see bare rocks with a deep
yellow-green soupy sea around them. Here and there slimy
things crawl on the rocks. There are explosions and upheavals
and great splashes in the sea as rocks fall into it. Great gushes of
steam break under your feet. The earth you stand on keeps
heaving, and you keep falling over. As you fall, you hurt your
legs and your buttocks. Everything around you seems to be
painful. Everywhere you step is too hot. You have no friends.
You are alone. You are angry with me for taking you here where
you have no control. Greasy, slimy things are crawling up your
legs. One of them is trying to get inside you. You pluck it off and
throw it away, but there are thousands and thousands of them
and eventually one goes inside your anus.

As it enters you, you know now that you have power, that
you can control everything around you. You send your mind
down, down into the base chakra. And from within it you
stamp on the ground, and the greasy, slimy things line up and
bow to you. You are strong. You glance at the sea and it moves
at your command. You glance at the land and it heaves in
response to your thoughts. Slowly at first, then more quickly,
you dance a crazy dance across the land that you own. As you
dance you smell the sulphur. You taste the rottenness of the
world you own. Yet it is yourself—and you are in control. Continue your dance now and understand your anger at the world,
for it is not pretty. And understand your desire to transcend it
and bring it into control.

In subsequent chakras the following instruction is omitted,
because it is the same for each in turn: Stay in petal meditation
for fifteen minutes. After fifteen minutes bring yourself back to
the present world. Be happy. Hug and kiss your friends and
review the results of your meditation.

Maithunic Marriage

Even if you are always working with the same partner, still you ritually marry each month for the next month.

After the base chakra meditation, members go through full and complete purifications. Being totally unbound and wearing no jewelry, they don a yellow and white sash. The sash leaves the genitalia naked and hangs down at the back in the form of a tail. This brings them back to the thought of the base chakra. It is animal, earthy, and primitive. The group comes together in a huddle in the center of the exercise room with males and females alternating. They enter into the most sacred part of the rite, for now the couples are going to become married for a month. The partners turn toward one another and each gently caresses the other's face. They usually murmur a few words of affection and ask the other to help them in the Great Task in the forthcoming month. A kiss is exchanged. They lie on the floor with the male on the female's right side. He lies on his left side and she turns her head so she can look into his eyes while she lies on her back. Gently he lifts her left leg over his legs and brings the lingam against the yoni by scissoring her right leg between his legs. Her left leg rests on his right hip. She reaches down and inserts the lingam into the yoni. They quietly lie in this position for 32 minutes. They make sexual movements. They play with each other, and they are encouraged to bring each other close to orgasm.

But orgasm should not occur. If either partner feels it is getting too close, all movement must cease, the breath is held, and the tongue is rolled back into the back of the throat. This rapidly brings the person back down from the orgasmic peak.

After 32 minutes, the couples rise and again join hands in the circle. They turn to one another and say words of marriage: "I swear by all I hold holy that I will help you in every way possible to develop in the forthcoming month." This is said in a normal voice and tone. In this way their sincerity is apparent. Hair rings are exchanged between the males and females; or if hair is not possible for some of the members, rings they have themselves carved from wood are exchanged.

They leave and sleep together. Loveplay is allowed but completion is still avoided.

There can be no thought at this time that the practice is in any way negative. Once you have completed this sacred ritual and have controlled your passions, once you have understood the power of creation, you know the path is opening for you.

ACTIVATING THE PELVIC CHAKRA

After overcoming and understanding the base chakra, you move upward[2] into other levels of awareness, entering the pelvic or sex chakra at midnight on the day of the Maithunic Marriage. When you approach the pelvic chakra from below, it is in its most raw reproductive mode. The goddess requires to be impregnated. Her whole mind and being are concentrated single-pointedly on getting a man to copulate with her so she can become pregnant. This chakra is approached at the end of the sexual fast and the Maithuna of the base chakra. It is not a love chakra; it is a lust chakra. The signposts for activating the pelvic chakra are as follows:

Symbol: Its symbol is the horns of a new moon. The tips of the crescent point upward, forming the worldwide symbol for the man cuckolded by his woman, who in her frustrated lust takes a lover.

Color: The color is vermilion—brilliant orange-red. It is the fierce anger of the person who has been cheated, and it is the red of virgin blood dripping from the yoni.

---

[2]Upward is a relative term. It may be along if you are reclining, or downward if you are standing on your head.

Emotion: The principal emotion of this chakra is said to be pitilessness, but that is not quite the feeling. There is a saying that a hard lingam has no conscience and will not be denied; this is the same sentiment applied to the female. The turned-on nymphomaniac is not going to be denied as she ruthlessly pursues her need. Because of her actions, there are tinges of other emotions in this chakra. She is suspicious and mistrustful: suspicious because of fear that she will be thwarted in her aim, and mistrustful of taking what is too freely offered. The emotions also apply to the male in heat.

Element: The element of this chakra is water, the first water appearing on the newly formed land. It contains many of the minerals of the land and indicates that new things will soon grow from the land. It tastes like sweat. Some say this water is indeed the sweat that is roused by furious copulation.

Sound: The sound of the chakra is that of a very angry sea pounding, pounding, pounding on the beach. Its rhythmic beating is the same as the beating together of bellies during hard copulation. The sound will not be denied. It is the sound of a force and a power which is beyond comprehension and beyond rational control.

The mantric sound is VA$\underline{M}$ repeated with the rhythm of the sea. The VA is very loud; the silent $\underline{M}$ tends to be short and very soft because it is the sound of the receding wave after the sea has hit the beach.

Animal: The animal associated with the chakra comes from the deep psyche. It is a hungry spider sitting in its web watching for a dainty morsel to be seized as it goes by. It is a female spider waiting for the male who will impregnate her—and then be eaten. Underneath, many men are afraid of a woman who comes to them demanding that her sexual needs be fulfilled. She is a threat to their very existence, because for centuries they have only performed when their lust was aroused. So he, too, turns to violent gluttonous fulfillment of his needs or dies. The

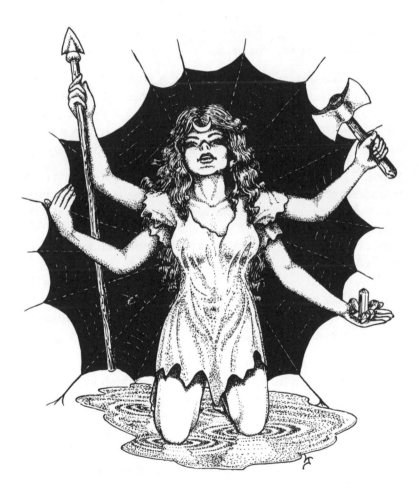

Figure 24. Rakini.

spider waits and watches its turn. It is going to eat, no matter what forces are brought against it.

Material: The material of the chakra is hard rock salt. It is a long, rather beautiful crystal, but the crystal cannot be seen until the outside edges are broken down. When it receives its opposite, water, it will totally melt away. It is in every living thing, and it is needed by every living thing. Yet in its present form it is too hard and rough to be used. It must be assimilated, its hardness mitigated, before it can be accepted.

Texture: The texture of the chakra is best appreciated by the thought of slightly damp sensitized skin. Imagine yourself to be sexually terribly deprived and at the same time in lust with a need beyond anything you have ever known before. Now a single touch on that most sensitive point at the tip of the lingam or the clitoris is the feel and the texture of this chakra.

Smell: The smell of the chakra is like that of bad fish. It is the odor of raw lust, the smell of dried semen combined with sweat. Perhaps it is best comprehended when you remember that "morning after" smell that occurs before bathing on the morning after a wild party. It is the smell that attracts the big black flies to the exposed lingam or yoni—flies that settle because the participants are too exhausted to raise a hand to brush them away.

Taste: The taste of the chakra is salty mucus in the very back of the throat. You feel as if you have eaten too much and it may come back at any moment, or that you are on a boat at sea and you are feeling ill and can taste the salt on your lips. It is the taste of expectation of fulfilled lust.

Goddess: The goddess of the chakra is Rakini (figure 24). Rakini is a strong and very female goddess. Her smooth, dusky skin is all-inviting. She is woman in her reproductive mode. She wants more children, and to get what she wants she puts on a gauzy, sensual robe that is slightly tattered from past encounters but nevertheless adds to her allure. Through it you can see she is as old as the world and as young as a virgin, and that she is on a lustful rampage. When fully understood, her drive hits you in the pit of the stomach. It is so basic, it is survival, and is in what might be described as the prehuman parts of the brain. For all her allure and all her emanations of rewarding femininity, beware: In her hands she carries weapons of destruction. If she is not satisfied, like the spider, she will unthinkingly destroy anything that gets in the way of her ultimate aim of being impregnated.

Ritual for Activating the
Pelvic Chakra

The members of the house gather in the exercise room after being sexually abstinent for several days and having controlled themselves in Maithuna. The yogis wear a blood-red loincloth of light cotton fabric. The yogins wear a light see-through blood-red robe. Each member has oiled the lower part of his or her belly with fish oil or oil in which fish has been steeped for several days. Everyone stands, males alternating with females, in a tight circle. To the hard VA of the VA$\underline{M}$ chant, they thrust their pelvises upward and inward toward the center of the circle and then slowly relax them on the $\underline{M}$. The pattern imitates the beating of the sea on the beach: the hard forward thrust as a wave hits and the smooth retreat as the water glides back down the sand into the sea.

The motion is kept up for several minutes until it is obvious that all members are ready and eager for sexual contact. The leading yogin breaks the circle. She grabs at the lingam of the yogi to her right and pumps it quite violently. The other yogins immediately follow her example. The yogis fall to the floor with the yogins on top of them. Each yogin tears off the yogi's loincloth and forces the yoni down over the lingam in a violent motion, so violent that in some houses lubricant is applied to the lingam and to the yoni before the ritual. Each yogin holds her body vertical; she does not lower herself onto the yogi in a loving manner. She moves violently upward and downward for eight strokes, then breaks off the encounter. Each yogin moves clockwise to the next yogi and treats him in the same way. At this stage no one reaches climax. The yogis are passive; the yogins remain ravening and violent.

Now in the second round of contacts each yogin becomes more cunning in her actions. She is more coy and more gentle. Now the yogi is rutting in need. When she approaches him, he throws her on her back and thrusts into her. She scratches and bites. He responds by kissing her violently while continuing the thrusts until he climaxes. But she is not yet satisfied; she wants it again. With all her feminine wiles she works on the lingam until it is hard again and he is inside her once more.

At this stage many houses allow the use of the whip to encourage and rouse the yogi. This is one of Rakini's weapons. She must have him again before the ritual ends. She can be as loving now as she wants, but she will not be denied.

The point of understanding of the chakra occurs at the instant before reaching the second climax. At this instant the yogi may try to withdraw, but the yogin forces continuation. It is in this attempted withdrawal and forced continuation that the chakra is finally entered. The spider has drained the mate.

Guided Meditation

This meditation occurs after the ritual. It is a stem lingam-yoni meditation. The first phase is to do a deep and complete meditation on the other gender's sexual equipment; in other words, the yogi meditates on the yoni and the yogin meditates on the lingam, strongly emphasizing nipples, clitoris, and lingam in an erected state. It starts with the state of erection that results from a long unfulfilled need for sexual satisfaction, and ends with the explosive orgasm. You can use the following meditation to help enter the chakra:

Come with me now and visualize, smell, taste, feel, and understand as you go along this path. You are on a path of velvet. It is smooth and dusky brown. You know it leads to completion. As you go along you see that you must pass the web of a giant spider that is about to mate. As you approach the spider's web encompasses you. It is warm yet dangerous. You find you can pass the web. You see the spider has consumed a male. It is warm. The dead spiders smell of fish. Though in some ways you are afraid to proceed, you are drawn onward as if someone had placed a fishhook in your guts and were pulling you along. As you are pulled along, the feeling in the pit of your stomach grows more urgent. The lingam and the yoni seem to grow. Now there is a live spider on the path. The lingam enters the spider's vagina. It is sucked and caressed. The spider's lingam enters the yoni and thrusts in. You are being sexually ravaged by a spider, and it is good. You enjoy it. You can feel how very soon now you will be reaching your peak. You are coming up to it. Each motion from the spider brings you closer.

Suddenly the spider dissolves and is no more—but you have not reached completion, and you are furiously frustrated. But the path goes on. Now ahead of you a beautiful woman and man wait. Yet as you approach there is a glass wall between you and them. You have to break the sheet of glass. You break through and couple with your ideal mate. Thrust is returned for thrust and the beat of the sea is in your head. It is beating, beating, beating. You have no control over your body. At this point you fully comprehend and enter the chakra.

ACTIVATING THE NAVEL CHAKRA

This chakra is the first in which the mind begins to control and direct the body. Whereas the first two chakras have drawn uninhibited, uncontrollable, subhuman, passionate, irrational responses from what is called the reptilian brain, now the mind is going to control and direct the body's activity. The mind has been totally shut off during the experience of the base chakra and the pelvic chakra, and it is repulsed by the body's activity. It is also confused, because it finds that part of itself enjoyed what the body was doing—contrary to everything you have ever been taught in the socializing process. "How can I allow myself to do those things—and what's more, enjoy them?" might be the question on which to meditate. The signposts for activating the navel chakra are as follows:

Symbol: The symbol of the chakra is a triangle with point upward. The base of the triangle represents the firm base and firm control which your mind thought it had over the body. The upward-thrusting point is the point on which you may destroy yourself, for it represents the uncontrolled urges and primal emotions which are barely held in check by the mind. The triangle is tall and slender when you first see it. Gradually its base widens out as the mind takes increasing control, but the point is always there. It is acknowledged; it is understood. At certain times as desire again engulfs you, you know that the triangle will become less stable and may approach a single vertical line that is totally unstable for some people.

The danger that every teacher fears in Tantra is inherent in this chakra. The total uninhibited enjoyment of the base and pelvic chakras can be constantly repeated and can become the alpha and omega of a person's practice. Yes, students go through the motions of the remaining chakras, for the search for bliss, but the only reason they do it is so that they can participate in rituals that require uninhibited behavior. If you have enjoyed the base and pelvic rituals and then leave the house to try to obtain the same enjoyment in the outside world, you may destroy yourself in the search. For in the house, the behavior is understood within its rightful context; whereas in the world the behavior is often proscribed. In most cases, the yogins are able to understand and control their emotions better than the yogis can (especially the younger ones). Tantra does not give you a set of commandments. Instead it is up to you to make your triangle as broadly based as you can—and also to allow it to become unstable when such instability is appropriate.

Color: The color of the chakra is blue and yellow. The blue of your spiritual aspiration is mixed with the dirty yellow of your baser instincts. The yellow turns the blue into green and spoils the color. When you first see the color, it is all green; but as you look at it and think about it and experience it, you are able to turn it more and more blue.

Emotion: The emotions of this chakra are a most complex mix of possessiveness, jealousy, and aversion. They start with a fear that you may never again be able to experience the pure pleasure that you got from the base and pelvic chakras. There is a possessiveness about you: You would like to totally own the person with whom you obtained the pleasurable sensations. Yet there is an aversion, a "Will you still respect me in the morning?" feeling; for you have let down all your barriers. You have shown the naked you to that person as to no one else. He or she knows you as no other person can. You are fearful that he or she will whisper to other people what your weaknesses are. You jealously watch your partner to make sure he or she won't give you away. You know in your heart of hearts that these feelings are assumed to be negative—that by having them you risk souring relations with the very person you want to possess sexually. At the same time the mind is making you feel disgusted with yourself for the body's uninhibited behavior. It is difficult to bring yourself to the level of maturity where you can forgive yourself for being so human.

To meditate on these emotions, it is best to examine possessiveness and jealousy in all their attributes, both negative and positive. The positive protective instinct can be contrasted with the negative ownership feeling. It is the slave-versus-idol and in some ways the virgin-whore conflict. Add to that the knowledge that you will seek this pleasure again, and you begin to comprehend the complex emotions of the chakra.

Element: The element of the chakra is represented by fire playing across water and fire eventually overcoming water. In the age-old swamp that rose from the sea, you saw land coming from water; then you saw water on the land. Now you see St. Elmo's fire: the bright beautiful flames rising from the rotting vegetation below the surface. The beautiful lotus grows best when it can absorb the muck and the filth—which are full of nutrients—below it. Your spiritual fire burns brightest when it can overcome the primitive pleasures of the body. Knowing the pleasure and overcoming it on a regular basis make the fire burn brightly. Having experienced the pleasure vicariously through reading about it or living it many centuries ago and then overcoming it does not give the fire the same brilliance, the same heat and intensity as does the regular repetition of real worldly pleasure.

Sound: The sound of the chakra is thunder: the dull thunder of primeval forces and primeval urges. It is ever present. The storm can blow up unexpectedly. The stronger the storm, the more powerful the thunder, the more brilliant the lightning, the more powerful becomes your will as you understand and comprehend it and move on.

The mantra of the thunder is RA<u>M</u>. The RA is deep in the chest. It is the lower pelvic thrust of thunder—boom. . .boom—that vibrates your whole universe.

Animal: The animal of the chakra is the ram. The shepherd knows that the ram is full of reproductive energy; that if there is nearby a ewe in heat the ram will batter his head mindlessly against the side of a cage trying to escape.

Material: The material of the chakra is burnished copper. It is beautiful in its polish. It gleams brightly. If you neglect it, though, it will become dull and green verdigris will spread across it, marring its surface. You can keep the copper shining brightly. You can keep the verdigris at bay. The mind can control the body. If you are disciplined, you will polish the copper regularly; if you do not fully understand the verdigris, you stop bothering to polish the copper—for to some the green verdigris is also beautiful. But you have learned to like the brightly polished copper better, and so you spend the time to polish and to remove blemishes.

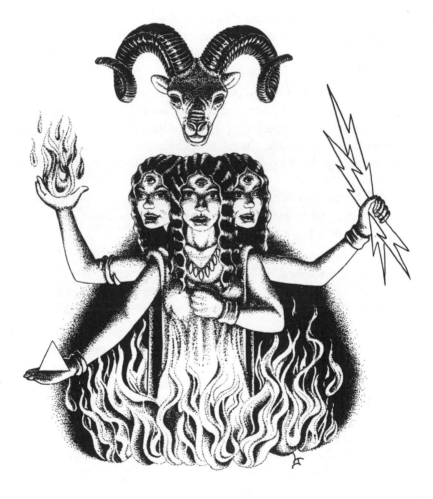

Figure 25.　Lakini.

Texture: The texture of the chakra is hard, vibrantly healthy skin. The skin over good tight buttocks or over a tight flat abdomen epitomizes this chakra. Think for a moment of the tight skin over a calf muscle. How quickly can that skin become loose if the muscle gets out of condition? The athlete with rippling muscles and beautiful skin has achieved this perfection by disciplined training. The athlete may be overdisciplined and overtrained, but the texture you are looking for here is that implied by tight skin over strong, controlled, moving muscle.

Smell: The smell of the chakra is the slightly acrid smell of sweat on a clean body. The basic smell is unpleasant, but somewhere in the smell the slight acridness gives a pleasant hint of work that has been done. This is not the smell of old sweaty dirty bodies; it is the honest smell of someone who has worked up a sweat in doing useful work and will shortly wash it away.

Taste: The taste of the chakra is a combination of opposites — cold, greasy mutton fat and sharp, astringent rosemary. To gain bodily nourishment, if you had nothing else to eat you could eat cold fat. It would be repulsive to you, but the taste could be more easily tolerated if at the same time you chewed rosemary leaves. Thus the combination of the herb and the fat gives you nourishment, just as the combination of the mind controlling the body gives you spiritual nourishment. The understanding that at any time you can control these primordial passions strengthens the spirit. You see the Tantric emphasis on not allowing the senses to atrophy or the pleasure gained from lustful behavior to be forgotten. In Tantra the senses are not atrophied; they are honed to piquant sensitivity. For overcoming the desire for something which is not very nice when you get it has no strengthening effect on the spirit. Only the overcoming of the desire for something that is very desirable strengthens the spirit.

Goddess: The goddess of the chakra is Lakini (see figure 25). She is a beautiful goddess with a dusky skin that promises smoldering sensual passion. Her naked body is covered with every imaginable jewel. Perhaps she is the concubine of a millionaire who has showered on her a fair portion of his wealth. She is most beautiful. Yet she covers herself and her jewels with a yellow robe. Her glancing eyes hold deep promise. Above those lustrous eyes she has a third eye in her forehead which is opening. You know that if you sink into her two mundane eyes the third eye will close, but if you please her with controlled behavior her third eye will open fully. Beware, though—for in her hands she holds thunderbolts—the deep uncontrolled passion of the storm is still with her. In another hand she holds the fire of the spirit, and you know that if she closes her hand she can extinguish the fire. As you come to know her, she will allow the fire to burn more brightly.

In addition to her four arms she has three heads. If you look closely at her heads you see that in one her mundane eyes are wide open and her third eye is almost closed, and in two others her mundane eyes are hooded and her third eye is more open. The three heads remind you (each in its own way) of your triangle of control.

Ritual for Activating the
Navel Chakra

In the house, the urgency of sexual lust after the period of abstinence has been partially satiated; needs are at a lower level. The hard edge of desire has been dulled. All enter the exercise room wearing blue loincloths; over the shoulders each wears a yellow transparent robe. They gather together in a tight circle with arms around one another's waist and begin the mantric chant. The yogis chant deeply and resonantly in the most basso profundo manner they can. The yogins chant in a soprano voice reaching the highest pitch they can. The chant is alternated: first the yogins and then the yogis. It is lightning and thunder mixed. As the yogis chant, the pelvises are thrust forward toward the center of the circle and withdrawn on the silent $\underline{M}$. As the yogins chant, they tilt their heads slightly backward without any exaggerated movement. When the group is really without any exaggerated movement. When the group is really into the chanting, you can feel the significance of each part of the chant. It becomes a very beautiful and very moving study in contrasts. The chant ends on the men's deep thunder.

The yogins turn invitingly and caressingly to their partners. They invite them to lie on their backs and to be caressed. The yogis oblige and are caressed. Gradually sexual desire is raised. The yogin mounts the yogi and her thrusts are sure, hard, and purposeful. He pulls her down onto him so that the breasts touch, and forcibly slows her motion until they are lying together coupled but motionless. Gently he withdraws from her. Each removes the other's robe. He lays her gently on her back and caresses her and kisses her. He brings the lingam close to the yoni. She reaches for him and urgently pulls him toward her. He resists the urgency and they make love gently and reach a simultaneous climax in which both express their love and appreciation of their partner.

At all times throughout the ceremony the mind controls. There is no frenzy or totally uncontrolled behavior.

Guided Meditation

After completing the ritual, sit in meditation in a close circle almost touching the other members of the house. Meditate first on the past. You can use the following guided meditation:

Imagine yourself going through the previous rituals. Start by getting involved in the hurting anger of the base chakra. Remember how you fought with one another and remember how you lost control, especially how you lost control in the frenzy of sexual activity in the pelvic chakra. Remember . . .

You are walking into a valley. As you go down into the valley you see beautiful people hurting one another, not only hitting and stabbing and punching, but also spitting and yelling obscenities. As you go deep into the valley you see animals that turn into human figures writhing in every imaginable form of

sexual congress. In some the women are on top; in others the
men are on top. In some the men are behind, doing sex like
dogs. In all their eyes are shut and their faces ecstatic with the
pleasure of their union.

You walk across the valley. You are both horrified by what
you see and fascinated by it. You cannot take your eyes off each
new scene. Now you begin to walk up out of the valley. As you
do, you see people caressing each other and making love in
beautiful surroundings in comfortable rooms. You are leaving
the smell of the valley behind. You can see the blue sky ahead of
you. Now you yourself meet with a lover and you begin to caress
and to make love. You come to beautiful, controlled completion, for although you could climax very quickly, you wait and
control yourself so that you climax at the same instant as your
lover. With the pleasure of it you blank out; then you awake to
find yourself back in the meditation room.

ACTIVATING THE HEART CHAKRA

The control that was exercised in the navel chakra to overcome
the primal urges of the reptilian brain is now complete. In some
ways this represents the death of desire; but in others it represents the total overcoming of desire by both the mind and the
spirit "I." "I" is now beginning to make its presence felt in the
mind; and since "I" is not of this world, as you approach "I" the
mind must firmly control desire. The signposts for activating the
heart chakra are as follows:

Symbol: The symbol of the chakra is the hexagram. If you look
closely at the hexagram, you see that it can be considered either
as two interlaced triangles or as six triangles fitted together. This
means that all the triangles of the navel chakra are brought
under control and combined into a symmetrical entity. Each
individual triangle represents one aspect of your awareness.
Thus your awareness through touch has the same size and shape

as your awareness by smell, by feel, or by any of the other senses. In other words, each sense and each emotion have the same weight in your awareness, and each is individually balanced and perfect. For each part of the triangle not only fits with its neighbor but is (in and of itself) balanced; for each of its three sides is of equal length.

Color: The color of the chakra is the lightning that you saw in the navel chakra, though it is no longer threatening. Instead its lustrous color pervades you. For "I's" divine fire is of a beautiful light purple color that shines with its own inner light. The closest comparison to the color is to think in terms of a beautiful light purple fluorescent paint.

Emotion: The feel of the chakra is one of relief at being able to overcome the baser emotions and cherishing the ultimate knowledge of how you did it. You are a great success. You want to go around the world telling everyone you are totally balanced and in control; yet the knowledge is so precious that you hug it tightly to yourself. When you see other people, you know you are better than they are, so you feel slightly arrogant. In the first flush of your success, you are in some ways not a nice person to know. Soon you will rise above the arrogance and will share your knowledge with others; but at this point and in this chakra you are still so full of yourself that you are unwilling to share.

Element: The smoke and hot air rise from the fire. With the experiences you have undergone you have been tested in the fire, and from the fire your spirit rises with confidence and power to take control of the fire. Thus the symbology of the air being formed from the fire is appropriate. Without fire there can be no smoke or air. If the smoke is not allowed to rise, the fire will be choked out. So the air must rise above the fire if the fire is to continue, and the spirit must rise above the body if the body is to serve its purpose. The body is only the temporary house of the spirit.

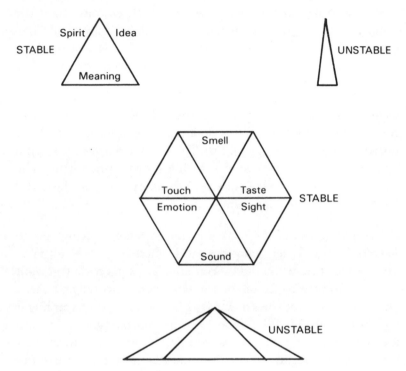

Figure 26.   The jewel in the heart.

Sound: The sound of the chakra is that of bells being rung hard and firmly and yet making no apparently recognizable tune. With careful attention and fine-tuned hearing, you eventually detect a pattern in the sound of the bells. This is a mathematical pattern, perhaps generated by an abstract program in a computer. Nowhere do you pick up a recognizable tune, yet the pattern makes sense, and you can tell that after a long time the random pattern repeats itself—just as life repeats itself, and your experiences in the Tantric cycle of the month repeat themselves.

The mantra of this sound is YA<u>M</u>. The sounds of the man-tra are extremely difficult. They must be varied not only in length, but also in intensity and in pitch. In a group, everyone starts with the same mantra. One person is selected to vary the rate of repetition; another is selected to vary the volume; and another is selected to vary the pitch. Each person must under-stand that he or she must come back to the beginning-point at regular intervals. Now imagine yourself listening to this group. There is no tune, but there is some mathematical order behind the mantra.

Animal: The animal of the chakra is the antelope. It is a very healthy animal but it is running away in startled fear from some unspecified attacker. As it runs effortlessly, its hide glistens and the muscles ripple along its flanks. Every so often it bounds over an obstacle. Soon it loses its fear and runs freely for the joy of running. The bounds grow higher until it is running and jump-ing in exuberant understanding of its life and its power over nature.

Material: The material of the chakra is sapphire. It has the hard firmness of a stone formed in the fire, but it has the beautiful light blue color of the spirit. It combines the perfection of the jewel with the color of your understanding. The sapphire is cut with triangular faces. As you look on it, you see that its outline is that of a hexagram. Yet the points of the triangles are raised; that is, each of the triangles has two long sides and a shorter base side (see figure 26). You know that the points can be dan-gerous; Yet because of its perfect symmetry and its color, instead of changing it, you will appreciate its underlying meaning.

Texture: The texture of the chakra is that of bone. Rub your finger across a bone and feel its grainy feel. Feel over the top of the joint. This is smoother. That fine graininess represents your wish to be in and of the world. The bone supports the frame of your body; it is the structure that carries your consciousness with it. The bone is a most necessary part of you, for dwelling

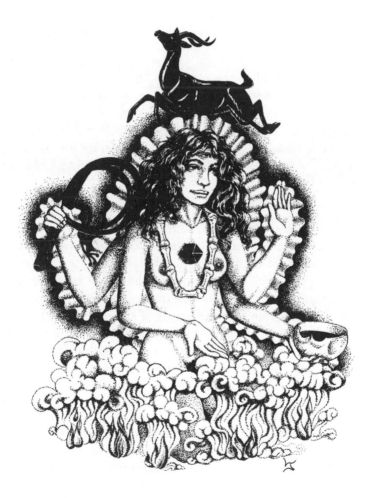

Figure 27.   Kakini.

within the cage of bones is the consciousness, the "I" which controls the mind which controls the action of the bones.

Smell: The smell of the chakra is the smell of fresh blood. It is a fairly light odor, yet one of terrible psychic importance, for the smell indicates the release of a spiritual being. The blood itself is part of the mundane body. Fresh blood reminds you that each being is mortal. The smell reminds you to pay attention to the spiritual part of yourself, for eventually only the spiritual part will remain.

Taste: The taste of the chakra is that of dark black, bitter chocolate. The world can be a trying and bitter place to live. You are often frustrated in the things you want to do, but once you understand this bitterness—once you fully comprehend how it affects you, once you can acknowledge that setbacks are an opportunity for growth and that pleasure of the world is also an opportunity for growth—then you can taste the full depth of chocolate and fully appreciate its subtle, complete flavor. If you let the world frustrate you or let it take you in lustful pleasure, you will never taste the chocolate—only the bitterness.

Goddess: The goddess of the chakra is Kakini (see figure 27). She is an attractive olive-skinned lady. She has three old eyes; each is equally open. She views the world from her vast experience. She has seen everything and she knows all the ways of the world. She has four arms and four hands. One of the hands makes the gesture of fearlessness. You must not fear her or the world. If you are not afraid, another hand tells you, she will grant you any boon you wish. This clearly shows that if you go out into the world and experience it, you will be rewarded with every sensual pleasure it has to offer.

Kakini holds a whip to remind you to pay attention to the development of your spirit instead of remaining only in the sensual world. If you do not pay attention to the spirit, she will goad you onward to this goal. In another hand she holds a cup made from a skull, containing the most exquisite wine of life you could ever imagine tasting. Drink from the cup the wine of life, remembering always that you will die. You are mortal. As yet another reminder of your mortality she wears a necklace of bones. Her spirit, too, is encircled in bones, just as your spirit is contained within your skeleton.

She is a lustrous goddess, shining with an inner light. Yet this turned-on nature is softened by the wine she has drunk from her cup. She understands sensual pleasure and she understands that even this can improve the brilliance of your inner life. But she stands ready to whip you to fulfill your destiny — while at the same time telling you to enjoy every pleasure you can find.

Ritual for Activating the Heart Chakra

For this ritual it is best for the exercise room to be equipped with black lights. The participants are garbed in white robes. Each dyadic couple comes in very softly. All stand and talk in whispers. At no selected time, but when all feel it is appropriate, they form a circle with such a circumference that each can reach to touch the fingertips of the next one in the circle. One person is selected to control each of the variable elements of the mantra — volume, pitch, and speed. The chanting begins. As the volume builds and the pitch drops, the participants gradually close the circle. As the volume decreases and the pitch rises, the circle is widened again. When it is done properly, the circle rhythmically opens and closes like the opening and closing of some seaplant under water or the yoni seeking a lingam. The patterned pulsing superimposes itself on the non-rhythmic mantra. When the circle is in and tight together, members are encouraged to stroke the hair and cheek of the person next to them. As they go apart they withdraw into themselves. They know that if they wish they can experience sexual pleasure, but they draw apart so that their spirits may understand that they are willing to forgo pleasure so the flame of spirit can be brightened.

When all feel the mantra has been chanted long enough, the person who is controlling it will naturally bring it back to the place from which it started. Now is the time for another Maithunic ritual.

Members lie in this Maithuna for a few moments enjoying each other and remembering the sensual pleasure they have shared together. Then they withdraw, sit separately, and go into meditation.

Guided Meditation

This is a meditation on the hexagram. Each triangle of the hexagram in turn is examined and meditated on. It is normal to start in the triangle of sight:

How well balanced is your triangle of sight? Visualize a limpid pool. If a rock is suddenly thrown into it, can you accept with equanimity the change in the surface of the water? It presents no threat to you. The suddenness of the change is like the change of mood of someone you are dealing with—abrupt, unexpected, and outside your control.

Now the pool is still again and you see reflected from its surface a beautiful naked lover who can fulfill your every wish. Gaze on the lover. Think of being fulfilled by the lover. Suddenly the surface clears and only trees are reflected in the pool. Again, how far out of balance did your thoughts and sight of a lover pull your balanced triangle of sight?

Move on now to your triangle of smell. You can smell roses: beautiful deep red roses. As you smell the roses, somebody dumps manure on their roots and it is not good manure. It is rotten manure that smells awful. When the manure has been absorbed by the roses, you smell the roses again. Now the scent of rose changes to the green, sharp smell of mint. After a moment this smell fades and the natural scent returns. How did these odors affect you? Were you able to comprehend them? Did you keep your triangle in balance?

Continue this exercise for each of the triangles, going in turn through taste, textural feeling, sound, and emotion. This is a long meditative cycle. It is difficult because your comprehension of smell, for instance, may not be as good as your comprehension of sight. Do not cheat in your meditation and express smell in terms of sight or vice versa. Try for pure meditation on the pure sense. For instance, don't do as one student did and say, "That tastes the way chloroform smells." Even though that is a perfectly logical description, it is in fact cheating in balanced meditation because you are converting one sense into another.

ACTIVATING THE THROAT CHAKRA

You are complete. You are balanced. You have overcome, understood, and controlled your sensual pleasures. You have achieved much—more than most people achieve in the whole of their lives. Yet you know there is more. You are not yet complete, for you have not comprehended the death of the spirit. You can understand mundane death. You can even accept the fact that the spirit will go on when the body is just a pile of bones. You must force yourself to go to higher levels of comprehension. It is difficult. You feel you have done enough. You are suspicious that those who urge you on know not of what they speak. Yet in your heart of hearts you must strive for completion. The signposts for activating the throat chakra are as follows:

Symbol: The symbol of the throat chakra is a circle in a flat plane. It is the circle of completion, the circle of understanding. Yet when you look carefully at it, you see that it is both a disk and a sphere. It is a multidimensioned, multifaceted object; and though you can comprehend the circle and see it as completion, it is not all that you can achieve. The sphere represents something beyond the disk. It is toward the sphere that you must strive.

Color: The color of the chakra is glistening light yellow. The easiest way to comprehend it is to cut a lemon in half and meditate on the glistening perfection of its fruit. It has symmetry, it is surrounded by a circle, it is contained within the white of its rind.

In the Tantric system, the light, lustrous, glistening yellow of the inside of the lemon is a higher color symbology in an upward progressive sense than that of the lustrous lightning of the heart chakra. In Western symbology, purple is often used to denote the highest levels of awareness. In Eastern symbology, a perfection of light is perhaps *all* light—which might be black or might be something else which is not black, but yet is a total absence of all colors. Perhaps that total absence is white.

Emotion: The overriding emotion in the throat chakra is understanding. It combines the mercy and the blessing of the goddess on you who strives to gain a higher understanding with the bittersweet knowledge of traveling this path—that you may lose what you have gained and when you move onward into the spiritual planes, you may never be able to return to the great pleasure you found at the physical levels. Thus the merciful blessing from the goddess combines with bitterness and even some annoyance because the total awareness of the mundane world is now regarded as merely the first few steps on the ladder.

Element: The element of the chakra is creation. Just as in the mundane world earth is the first element created, so now you are creating life from the air that rose from the fire. It is the first step on the second turn of the spiral. It has a relationship to earth, in that objects are created from the materials in earth; yet it is so far above earth that it's difficult to comprehend.

Sound: The sound of the chakra is that of the flute as it is played in upward scales. These are sounds produced from the breath of life. They are gentle, soothing, reassuring sounds, leading you onward and upward. The mantra is HAM. It is sounded in the reverse manner from normal mantras. The HA sound starts

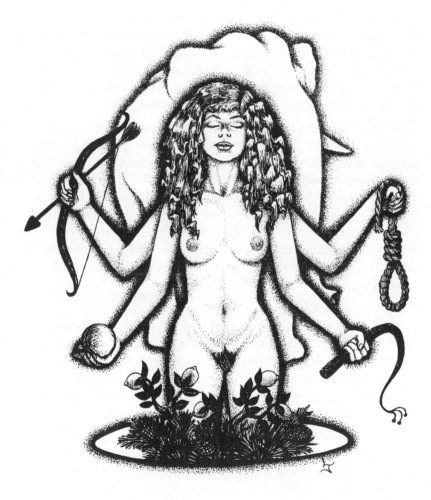

Figure 28.   Shakini.

very low and gains in power as it is pronounced so that the A overpowers the H and the silent M̲ vibration is louder than in most mantras, leading you upward from the low HA to the high M̲.

Animal: The animal of the chakra is the sacred white elephant standing alone and alert. You must approach it very carefully, for it still has many negative feelings toward the world and toward people who try to control it. It knows its own power. It is afraid of nothing in this world. Yet it is still unsure of itself—and it is still dangerous. If it is roused in the wrong way, it will fly into a rage and will be uncontrollable. It is a beautiful animal that anyone would love to own and to tame. And your task is set for you—it is the owning and taming of your own internal sacred white elephant.

Material: The material of the chakra is silver: a precious metal that can be molded to many shapes. The molding is done with comparative ease. Yet as silver is molded and shaped, it can lose its shine, can become black and dull. As you mold the silver of your spirit, you must forever be wary that it retain its lustrous untarnished silverness.

Texture: The texture of the chakra is the feeling you get when you gently stroke corduroy. When you softly stroke it along its ridges you have sensual feelings of pleasure and you know that you could stroke forever in that direction. You continue to enjoy it as you stroke it. Suddenly your hand is pushed across the cord and you feel the roughness of the ridges. If you resist, your fingertips are forced down into the cloth and the ridges become very rough. If you do not resist, you can brush lightly across the ridges and then continue to stroke along a new ridge of the corduroy. You find it is just as pleasant to stroke the corduroy at a higher level as it was at a lower level. You need not have resisted the push that carried you across the ridges.

Smell: The odor of the chakra is that of lemon or of an open pine forest. These are clean, astringent smells—smells you associate with new beginnings, with spring-cleaning the house, with getting out alone in the deep vastness of a pine forest. You know you have cleaned your own house. You know you are in balance. You know that "I" controls "Me" who controls the body. You have set the house of your body in order, and from that firm base you can move on.

Taste: The taste of the chakra is that of honey-sweetened lemon. There is a hint of bitterness here, but the honey overcomes it. You know that in the pure form the lemon is sour, but the honey that has been added to encourage your continuing has made it a very pleasant taste indeed—a taste you want to return to because it promises that future tastes will be even more pleasant.

Goddess: Shakini is the pale goddess of the chakra (see figure 28). She knows the whole world and everything in it. Her purpose is to drive you on. She has her whip ready and will not hesitate to use it on you. If you resist her will, she will use the bow and arrow that she holds in her other hands, or even the noose. For by using these weapons she can surely send you on the path from which no return is possible; and she will not hesitate to kill you if you do not proceed along the upward path.

Yet for all her threatening aspect, she is a friendly goddess; she is mercy personified. If you falter, she will help you. If you fail, she will be merciful. If you do not attempt the path, though, she will kill you, for you must aspire to higher things or die in the attempt.

Ritual for Activating the
Throat Chakra

The members of the house come to the meeting in normal, clean, everyday clothing that represents work garb, wearing no jewelry. Each brings a lemon and a small quantity of honey. They place all this in the center of a circle. All stand with hands joined. They chant the mantra with its special rising cadence.

Usually eight or twelve chants serve to tune everyone's mind in to the ritual that is about to take place. After the chant, the circle is broken and each dyadic pair goes through the following sequence. First, the yogin does it to the yogi; then the yogi does it to the yogin.

The yogin places around the yogi's throat a thin piece of linen fabric. He clenches both fists above his head in a hard, hard clench. She tightens the fabric around his throat. When he has had enough, he unclenches his fists. This is not a matter of either trying to strangle him or his being so macho that he wishes to feel pain in his throat before he unclenches his fists. The throat is a delicate mechanism, and even a light pressure may damage it. When there is pressure from the linen, the yogi must immediately unclench his fists. This is a symbolic ritual, not a test of endurance. After the role reversal, the yogi clenches his fists above his head and the yogin beats him with a whip, using very light strokes. The yogi should immediately unclench his fists. Then he again clenches his fists and unclenches them in response to the very gentlest stroking of his cheek by the yogin. In the first part, he is admitting that he will let go the world if he is faced with death. In the second part, he is admitting he will let go the world if he is beaten into it. In the third part he agrees to follow the path after only the gentlest persuasion.

For the final part of the ritual, the members gather around the pile of lemons and the little pots of honey. Each lemon is cut in half. Each participant sucks juice from one half of the lemon; then each takes one teaspoonful of honey. The lemon juice is squeezed out into an earthenware pot and the remaining honey is added to it. The mixture is carefully blended. Each member stirs the pot with a wooden spoon. Some of the liquid from the pot is decanted into a silver chalice. Each member smells and tastes the liquid. The nectar of the gods (the honey) has been mixed with the bitter knowledge of the world (the lemon juice), and the combination is better than the bitterness of the lemon or the sweetness of honey alone.

Guided Meditation

For this meditation, it is often helpful at first to use a crystal ball. Later in your development, imagine a crystal ball resting in your hands as you sit in meditation.

Look at the ball and notice its roundness. Think of your knowledge and how complete it is, and how it encircles you and guides all your actions:

Within the ball there is a misty light. Come with me now down into that mistiness.

We are on a path carved in a spiral shape up the side of a cliff. Part of the path is inside the cliff, and part of the path is outside. This is a very unusual cliff—its upper part is clothed in glass. The glass starts with no color and as it proceeds down the cliff it gradually becomes tinged with purple. Sunlight is reflected from the cliff. Every time you come out of the cliff on the path as you spiral upward along it you see new and more beautiful colors and hear sounds that are ever lighter, sounds that beckon you onward. It would be easy to turn around and slide back down the path and enjoy yourself sporting in the forest below, for people are down there and you can dimly hear their shouts of joy and party laughter above the beckoning music. In fact you turn and start back down. But you are stopped by an awesome female figure who threatens you with death unless you proceed. So reluctantly you turn and carry on—perhaps a little wearily—up your path. You are happy to have made the decision, but a little bitter that it was a decision you could not avoid. Gradually you reach ever higher. As you spiral upward, you find that the path inside the mountain is now light, even though it does not quite have the light of the path when it leaves the cliff face. Now you are proceeding with the quiet assurance that you will find and explore new and unknown realms, and that the effort you are making is well worth the small sacrifice of not being at the party.

Meditate now on this thought: You are unique. You are learning and progressing past those who are enjoying themselves at the party. After ten minutes or so of meditation, return, quietly walking down the path. The fearful goddess who forced you to move upward welcomes you and congratulates you and kisses and caresses you. She assures you that you will have more fun now at the party than you would have had if you had not attempted to scale the height.

ACTIVATING THE BROW CHAKRA

The greatest challenge to Western practitioners in comprehending the very high spiritual chakras is that the sexual symbology continues into them. Many Westerners cannot transcend the physical feelings of pleasure and completion that come from sexual activities to gain the spiritual significance and understanding that are in each chakra.

In the brow chakra the goddess first meets Shiva. At this stage he is still a dull god and he is still into mundane things of this world. She is so happy finally to meet someone who is her equal that she joins with him, not just sexually, but mentally and spiritually. It is a chakra of completion—the yin and the yang. At this point the three channels of the body come together: The Ida, the Pingala, and the Chitrini are all joined at this one point in space—and for a short interval in time a star bursts in space. The signposts for activating the brow chakra are as follows:

Symbol: The symbol of the chakra is an hourglass through the neck of which you must pass. It signifies the transition from the mundane to the spiritual, for this chakra is the "I" chakra. "I" is the spiritual being that controls "Me" that controls the mundane body. The hourglass symbol is combined with that of the erect lingam. Often in the pictures you can see semen suspended above the lingam, which has been ejaculated from it only moments before. The meaning is clear: This is creation in its pure form. The creation of life passes through the hourglass of the yoni and leaves the mundane behind. At the instant of orgasm and in the peace that follows, there is the total feeling of completeness, of satisfaction. From the goddess's point of view, she has been impregnated and fulfilled.

Color: The color of the chakra is brilliant, pure white. The god and the goddess are both purified by their completion. It is the whiteness of fresh live seminal fluid representing creation in its pure form.

Emotion: The overriding emotion of the chakra is completeness. The only satisfactory way of explaining it is to say that it is like the moment after orgasm while you are still firmly intertwined with your lover. The yoni is still vibrant and pulsing and the lingam, still erect, is totally and deeply contained within the yoni. You are one with your lover. You have both achieved your aim. Now is the time for patience, while the creation that you have formed grows and brings forth new life.

Element: The element of the chakra is life force. This is a superior form of water. New life has been formed, and already contains within it a tiny spirit. The awareness of this new spirit that is the result of creation is the element of this chakra. Those who see auras see a vibration of this type around women who are pregnant.

Sound: The sound of the chakra is very gentle and peaceful. The turmoil is over. You are complete and ready to go on. Instead of the beating of a bell, you hear its gentle stroking. It is a soft sound like the stroking of a lady's cheek, yet it is vibrant with the meaning of life, for it is the sound of the beginning of life. You can hear the resonance of the bell and you know it will become louder until you can fully hear and comprehend it.

The mantra of the chakra is the mantra of life—the O<u>M</u>. It is sounded softly, softly, softly. It will not be denied, for the silent <u>M</u> persists.

Animal: The animal image of the chakra is the coupled man and woman. They are coupled so their bodies form a yin-yang. In the last few centuries there has been a move away from this animal toward the tiny seedling of a flowering tree. The tree has been planted and little shoots are beginning to turn green. Everyone recognizes that this tiny seedling contains the thrusting power of life. If it is placed under a stone, it will lift and break the stone, for it is life itself.

Material: The material most associated with the chakra is a drop of living crystal-pure water or new seminal fluid. It is never static; it is always moving. All life needs this material, for without it everything dies. The sperm is contained in liquid. The egg is nurtured in liquid. So the element is more than just water itself, it is water containing nutrients. It is also (most importantly) the faint mist that rises from the water that will carry you onward and upward.

Texture: The feeling and texture of the chakra is that of gently, lightly stroking very clean hair. The hair is very fine. It is young and alive. But if you stroke it heavily you change the feeling to one of a rough-textured material that brings you down from the chakra. The touch is so light that it is hardly felt, just as at the moment of fertilization the egg has hardly changed, but you know that the boundless life energy is within it.

Smell: The young baby after a bath and before being powdered with a perfumed talc represents the odor of the chakra. It is the odor of life. It is the odor of warm newness and cuddly freshness. Small farm animals have this odor, when they are kept in clean dry stalls.

Taste: The taste of an apple just picked, still warm from the tree, is the cleanest freshest taste you can find. This is not a tart apple but a sweet one that has a very light taste in the mouth. Yet it is warm and firm. Do not chew on your apple. Savor its warmth, freshness, and newness.

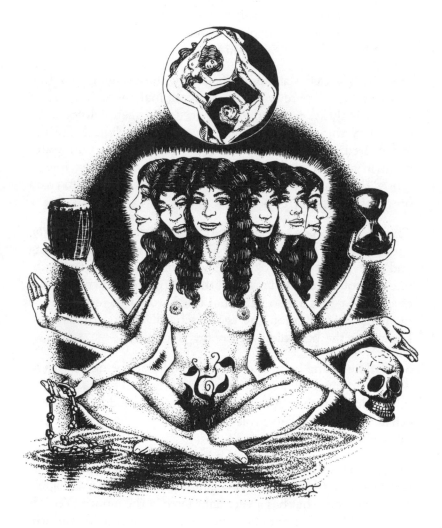

Figure 29.   Shakti.

Goddess: The goddess of the chakra is Shakti (figure 29). She is white. She is somewhat plump. She is the Shakti who has been refined from the goddesses of all the lower chakras. She has overcome all her driving desires and she has received what she wants. She smiles very contentedly. She knows that she contains the seed of new life.

Shakti has six heads so she may watch in every direction. In addition to the four cardinal directions, she also looks up and down to guard the new life within her. In her hands she holds a cord on which she counts the number of new lives coming into the world every day. She contemplates this wonder of new life and shows it to the world so it, too, may understand. She has a drum, which she gently strokes and beats with the slow controlled measure of life itself. She has a skull to remind you once more of your mortality and that you must create new life before you leave this plane of existence. After you have created new life, Shakti will grant you the boon of understanding spiritual life.

In some ways this goddess is complacent; in others she is a representation of total, ultimate passion, for she contains all the goddesses that were, are, and will be.

Ritual for Activating the Brow Chakra

This ritual requires that each member wear five robes, each of a different color, one on top of the other, to the exercise room. The colors represent the chakras that have been overcome in coming to this place. The yogis are hooded. The outermost hooded garment represents the base chakra, and the garments progressively represent the other chakras as you come up through them.

The leading yogin of the house carries a drum, which she gently strokes. One of the yogis carries a bell, which he gently strokes. All intone OM quite softly. Each yogin goes to a yogi and pulls off his hood. She expresses surprise and pleasure at seeing him. As they continue to make the sound of OM, they gently take from each other their outermost garment and put them into a symbolic fire. (Nowadays this can be a trash can. All that is required is that the symbol of leaving this level behind is clearly understood.) The OM grows slightly louder as they remove the next garment, and louder again as they remove the next garment. The speed and intensity of OM are increasing. They gently stroke each other's hair. Then they gently stroke the nape of the neck. They begin very gently and lightly to stroke the lingam and the yoni. When the last garment is removed, the OM is very loud. The yogi mounts the yogin and she pulls the lingam into herself, reaching down for the buttocks and firmly pulling the yogi down onto her while she lotuses upward to receive him. Full copulation occurs. It must be a firm and satisfying experience for both participants.

Everyone realizes that fertilization is not likely to occur at this copulation, but at the instant of mutual orgasm, the image of new life in its lustrous whiteness, its warmth and pinkness, must be held by both partners. They place their foreheads together at this instant and do their best to send their minds from one forehead into the other, to meld them and send them as a melded mind on upward. This mind-melding and upward transcendence of the body occur while the partners consciously maintain lingam and yoni fully joined. As the mind-melding occurs, the soft OM is repeated and the vibrations from the silent M are transmitted through the foreheads between the yogi and the yogin.

When they both get into this vibratory state, they often pass out and leave their bodies. This transcendence is the desired result of the ritual. Some participants find that if they lie side by side with foreheads touching and arms intertwined they can more easily transcend their bodies. Of course this position is fully approved.

Guided Meditation

This meditation is done in a hot bath or in the house as a group in the hot tub, immediately after a fulfilling orgasm. If it can be arranged, the room is dark and a single tiny point of white light is illuminated above the tub:

You are small, small, small. You are enveloped in warm moist affection. It is dark in here. Many passages lead in all directions. In the distance you can hear the quiet hum of life. Perhaps it sounds like the stroking of bells. A gentle vibration underlies everything. You look at yourself and you are white, yet you are full of life. You are content. There are many souls here. You are all friends. Slowly the vibrations become stronger, beckoning you to follow a spiral path through a cave which twists and turns around. As you follow the cave, you see that you are being pushed and pulled along by hundreds of your friends, and you in your turn are helping them along.

Suddenly the cave straightens out into a long smooth passage. Your excitement increases. You rush along the passage and suddenly break through into a new and different place of light where steam rises to a golden dome. Here you see someone whom you seem to have known, though you have never met. It is obvious that this is the other half of yourself. To live you must join with the other half, so you joyfully go forward and meld with this opposite being. At the point of melding all becomes still. There is no more hurry. There is no more vibration. You are one.

You rise now, floating gently upward, following the steam as it rises. You go toward a brilliant golden light. You see that together you must pass through the narrow neck of an hourglass. The glass is lustrous white. There are fine threads along its sides that you can slide up. It smells of dawn. It has the feel of dew on grass, yet it is warm and welcoming. You pass through the hourglass and go toward the light.

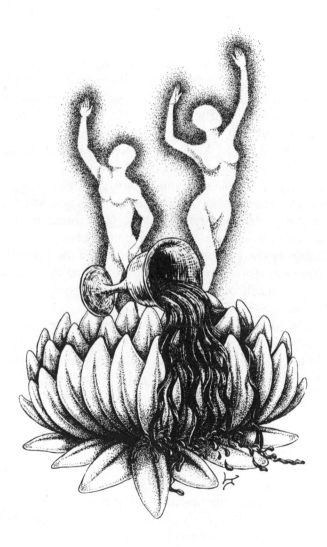

Figure 30.   The Crown.

Drift now toward the light. Let the thoughts come to you. Do not try to become one with the oneness. Let what will happen, happen. As the water cools, it brings you into yourself, but it cools so slowly that you come back down into it very slowly.

And now regretfully you separate with much pain from your Self and rejoin the mundane body.

ACTIVATING THE CROWN CHAKRA

The crown chakra is sometimes called the thousand-petaled lotus; at other times it is called the secret chakra. (See figure 30.) This is the secret beyond secret, for although all chakras are considered secret, the crown is the secret chakra of the chakras. At the brow chakra the threads of your mundane being—the Ida, Pingala, and Chitrini—have first coalesced and then separated enough to support "I." You are suspended floating between the three threads, touching none of them.

You are full of knowledge of the world. You have understood every sensual pleasure and every emotion. When you add one more drop to the container of your knowledge, it will burst; and in bursting it will propel you forward and out of these worldly things. You have in your mind many different thoughts. Each of them connects you to the mundane world; every thought engenders in you some kind of emotional response. You cannot view a scene in the world without affecting it in a subtle way. Even if you take no physical action, still by viewing the scene you have thoughts about it. The thoughts will travel out and affect the participants.

To comprehend and to pass into the secret chakra, you must be able to view any scene, from utmost sensuality to grossest depravity, without its having the least effect on you. Only with this total equanimity can you overcome the world and travel into the secret chakra. If you view some scene that is very negative, one which calls for action, you must not be affected by the scene or by the actions you should take.[3] The signposts for activating the crown chakra are as follows:

Symbol: The symbol of the chakra is the thousand-petaled lotus. Within the lotus you can see a cup emptying out a liquid that falls in infinitely fine streams, each of a different color. You are giving up all the things of this world—releasing them. In your mind you think of sensual and other pleasures, but as you think of them, your mind holds you still and emotionless.

Color: The color of the chakra is the color of light itself. In some ways light has no color, yet in other ways it contains all colors. Light can be either brilliant or dim. The physicists tell us it can be both a particle and a wave motion. It is this indefinable "light" color that you must strive to understand to comprehend the color of the chakra.

Emotion: The emotion of the chakra is timeless meditation that will lead to rapture. Nothing will disturb you. Time is available for everything you want to do. There is an agelessness about this—a timelessness—a feeling that you have been here before, perhaps a million years ago.

Element: The element is spirit from life force. The element of the chakra is in fact "I," your Self, your spirit. It is the divine force— if it can be called a force—that is the real you. After you have stripped away the body and the mind, underneath is the timeless piece of you, the "I," which never perishes. The unimaginable substance from which "I" is actually made is the element of this chakra.

---

[3]This yogic thought is very good advice for dealing with the mundane world. If you let your emotions become involved in your deeds, you will be unable to think clearly or act objectively. Even when you display emotions like anger, they must not make you angry and they must be completely under your command. From anger you must be able immediately to change into cold, hard objectivity.

Sound: The sound of the chakra is almost unheard. It is best likened to the sound that hot air might make when it rises on a very still day. It is the sound that you can hear only with the inner ear.

The mantra is still the sacred OM, but now the OM is made at so high a pitch that it cannot be heard by the physical ear. The only thing that you can imagine you hear is the movement of the mouth and tongue and the vibration of the head as the silent M is sounded. In making this OM, the mouth is opened, the tongue is moved, and the silent M inaudibly vibrates in the ethers.

Animal: The living being of the chakra is the sacred thousand-petaled lotus. Its petals have every possible color, shade, and hue imaginable. All the colors and shades are alive. As you look at each individual color and shade, they take you beyond every mundane color and shade and into new levels of awareness of color.

Although the chakra has color and sound, it has no taste, feeling, or smell, because these characteristics are traditionally considered to be too much connected with the mundane world to be appropriate. If a taste were to be assigned, it would be the taste of Nothing. If a smell were to be assigned, it would be the smell of Nothingness.

There is no further guidance for this chakra because the path is different for each individual and cannot be described in words—if it is described, you might see it as the guru says it is.

We have not attempted to give you a ritual or a guided meditation for the Crown. The territory is so variable that if you carry into it preconceived ideas, they will make feelings and pictures that solidify Nothing into Something. Contemplate the pictorial representation. It may help you on your path. Then try the standard stem and petal meditations without a ritual in between. People who spend many hours in sensory-deprivation

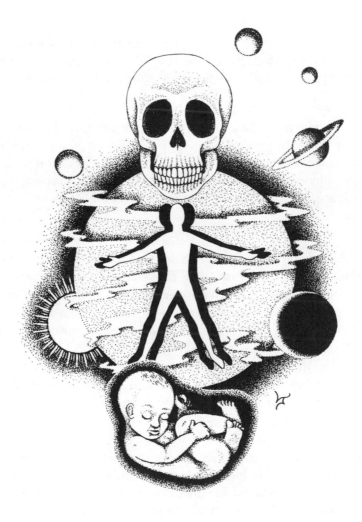

Figure 31.　Beyond.

tanks without an outside schedule pushing them seem able to comprehend part of this chakra.

BEYOND THE SECRET CHAKRA

It is possible for even the dullest of minds to have some comprehension of the secret chakra. Beyond the secret chakra lies the realm of Singularity. Into this realm you must venture by yourself. It is the ultimate aim of this guru that you do in fact go through the secret chakra and learn the ultimate truth.

As you may imagine, the symbology and signposts for the chakra beyond the secret chakra are both non-existent and totally existent. Every single microorganism—every single tiny blade of grass—contains the secret of the chakra beyond. Yet the secret is also in the emptiness of space. It is in life—it is in death. It is everywhere—it is nowhere. In simplistic terms it may be called the Void of Creation and it can be given attributes, like Everything, Anything, and Nothing. It is the place where "I" rejoins the "All" and surrenders its individuality. It is the place of the ultimate sacrifice. It is the mother from whom you came. It is the father to whom you will return. To get into it is the purpose of the Kundalini Circle. The whole message and secret behind the raising of the serpent power is in the fact that you must rush through the other chakras knowing them instantly as they occur but with a powerful upward thrust so that you will burst through the secret chakra into the one Beyond. (See figure 31.)

The Path Beyond the Secret Chakra

As the full moon approaches and passes, so a suppressed air of excitement pervades the house; for at midnight on the day of full moon the great Kundalini Circle begins. Complex hormonal changes have already occurred in the practitioners; and during the Kundalini Circles further changes will take place that make it progressively easier to overcome the body and leave it behind, then to leave the mind behind, and then to allow the spirit to meld with the Singularity. Refer to page 127 for the mechanical details of the circle. Each circle takes two hours and eight minutes.

Usually you are with your dyadic partner in the first circle. In the second circle you work with the person to whom you will be married next on the roster, and in the third circle with the next partner. In houses with only one or two couples, partners repeat quite rapidly. In a large house the full circle is not considered complete until every possible combination of partners has occurred.

In the first two circles smoky blue robes are worn. After eating, the members come together in a circle sitting on the floor very close to one another. In some groups, the females reach out and touch the very tip of the lingam and the males touch the clitoris. In this position they sound an OM of the small bells and everyone concentrates on someone who is far away. Usually this is an individual thought transference between a member of the group and (for instance) a parent or a child. Members quietly send thoughts of well-being and try to contact the person to find out what is going on in his or her life.

The ritual proceeds around the Kundalini Circle (page 127). Then the group again meets wearing their smoky-blue robes. Now a group telepathic communication is tried, usually of a healing nature. After the second circle is complete, members don long, flowing robes of a beautiful silver-gray. The group stands for the ritual. Sometimes recorded flute music is played while all listen quietly. They are full of love one for another, and their chant signifies this mutual loving feeling. After another circle is completed, members wear the same silver robes and repeat the same chant.

When the fourth circle is completed, all robes are laid aside. Now they sit separately in deep meditation remembering the chakra that has been passed. A quiet OM, the OM of the silver chains, is sometimes done. Some will gain Nirvana and a blissful state at the end of the fourth circle, though many will need more circles. Most houses will usually limit the circles to eight, saying that if the member has not gained enlightenment by that time, he or she must try for it the following month. But the scriptures define no limit; and if some members of the house wish to go on trying, there is no restriction on it.

Do not expect to reach the blissful state in your first month or two in the work. You may need many months to reach it. Once it is reached and the chakra is fully understood, as the months progress and the circles continue, it becomes easier and easier to get into this chakra. You should never willingly try to do it in less than four circles; for once you have reached it, it is very difficult to come back down and complete another circle to help a partner into bliss. Many houses find that their members of longer standing have to form their Kundalini Circle separately from the newer members because they know how to ride the path and it slows them down too much if they are constantly forced into doing eight or more circles for the sake of those of lesser development.

The circles should be continued for as long as possible for the benefit of those who don't make it; but for the benefit of those who have made it, they have to be realistically curtailed.

CHAPTER

NINE

Descending the Chakras:
Illumination

AS YOU ASCENDED through the chakras, you understood and overcame your various bodily appetites. You did not reject them or suppress them, but you indulged them in a controlled manner so you could comprehend the whole of your character. From that wholeness of comprehension, you were able to leave your mundane body and gain spiritual illumination. You got on a high which is beyond any high you had previously known, and you are confident that you can reach that high or an even higher one in future months.

Coming back down in a controlled way is just as important as reaching upward; for if you do not come down, you may be inclined to commit suicide or do yourself some mental injury so that you may simply stay in your Nirvanic tranquility. You must come down to re-gather your forces so that next time you can start your journey with more knowledge and more illumination and can reach higher.

As with ascending the chakras, you are allowed two days to master each descending step and its chakra. Follow the instructions on pages 155–157 for meditations to do before and after each ritual.

ILLUMINATING THE CROWN CHAKRA

As you come back down the chakra keeping the steps in time with figure 17 on page 123, your WILL illuminates them. The illumination is represented by the various forms of Shiva, who is now brilliantly illuminated. In all his forms the god is more restrained, more spiritual than his female counterparts, whom you met as you ascended through the chakras.

Remember that Tantra recognizes that all the power in the world stems from life itself – and the Keeper of Life is the female, not the male. The male is an occasional necessary appendage to the dynamic, emotional, lustful attributes of Mother Nature. *She* is the primal moving force behind everything. At first it seems that assigning the spiritual aspects to the male and the earth aspects to the female makes the religion chauvinistic. You must realize that in the day of Tantra's prime, fertility held the key to the future: not only fertility of the race itself, but also the fertility of the crops and fields. Mother Nature was and is a dynamic, unimaginable force, the most powerful force in the universe. Only after she is satisfied can spirituality be approached.

Tantrists live in this world. They are very dependent on Mother Nature to fulfill the sensual pleasure aspect of their control and belief system. Therefore she is looked after first. She must be looked after before illumination can occur.

You are a brilliantly illuminated being. You have had an experience which will stay with you the rest of your life. The experience has shattered many of your preconceived notions and feelings about reality. You are a being of light, a Shining One. You are ready to be reintegrated with your body, but you are existing as a spirit entity in the crown chakra. You are not yet re-integrated with your body – controlling it, you are not even contemplating being re-integrated. Instead you are "I," the ruler and owner of a body that has been assigned to you. Right now you are a separate, individual, complete entity. You can communicate with the mundane body and hear and see everything it sees. Sadly you know you must come down, and you decide to bring some of your joy and illumination with you. As each chakra is approached, remember that after the signposts you must do a stem meditation on them before proceeding in the ritual. The signposts for illuminating the crown chakra are as follows:

Symbol: There is a container in which "I" seems to fit. It is a beautiful crystal chalice. "I" is contained within it. It is so brilliantly illuminated you cannot bear to look directly at it. Your cup is full. You understand everything.

Color: The color of the chakra is the color that would produce a brilliant bluish-white light in a crystal cup. It is the essence of light itself.

Emotion: The emotion of the chakra is humility. You have been part of something which is so much greater than yourself that you are humble and grateful to the Singularity for having momentarily been a part of It. Another emotion is often mixed in—the sense of awe. This is not the piety or awe of downtrodden masses—it is the awe of someone who has had an ultimate experience and can remember that he or she is part of the Eternal One.

Element: The element is the substance of spirit. As you return from the void of the chakra Beyond, you have changed from nothingness into "I," the eternal spirit. The essence of the chakra is therefore spirit matter.

Sound: The sound of the chakra downward is that of the sacred O<u>M</u> sounded without sound. That is, the mouth is opened, the tongue is moved, and the body vibrates in imagination on the silent <u>M</u>. It is sounded with illumination and with knowledge, at such a high pitch that it cannot be heard. That is the difference between it and a very similar sound made as you approach the chakra from below. The sound now is luminous; it is a living sound.

Animal: The being in this chakra is the thousand-petaled lotus. Its leaves contain every color and every shade, and now those leaves glow with their own inner illumination, as if a million-watt light bulb had been lit inside the lotus. You can see the glow from the leaves and the leaves interpose themselves between the brilliance of the light and your eyes. Only this fact allows you to know you have already been through the light and that the lotus is full of the nectar of your knowledge. Now quietly and reverently do your standard stem and petal meditation on the chakra. No ritual or guidance is given here because the guru has not found one appropriate to this level that is suitable for all practitioners.

ILLUMINATING THE BROW CHAKRA

As you reenter the brow chakra from above, you bring new knowledge, new light, and illumination. You do not want to return. You have had a good vacation from the cares and pressures of the mundane body, and you are well rested. You know you must return, but you are sorrowful that you must. Only in returning from vacation can you earn some more money so you can go on vacation again. The signposts for illuminating the brow chakra are as follows:

Symbol: The symbol of the chakra is two tiny petals on a small plant or lotus. It can also be the first blossom of spring on a flowering tree. The new life you formed as you reached upward is beginning to gain understanding, and the understanding that you brought back from the place beyond the Crown will help it to grow and become more beautiful.

Color: The color of the chakra is white. Whereas the color from below was tinged with the pinkness of new life, now it appears to be tinged very slightly yellow; for you have progressed beyond the lustrousness of pure white. You understand that this whiteness is now more beautiful than it was when you approached it from below, for you understand whiteness in its full enormity. Any whiteness of this world is necessarily tinged with the world, and it can never be as pure to you again as it was before you achieved oneness.

Emotion: The overriding emotion of the chakra is now sorrow. You were at the place of oneness, totally melded with the "That-ness" of understanding. Now you must leave that place. To a woman, it is as if she had lost her dearest child. To a man, it is as if the most cherished wife had passed on. You know that the spirits have gone onward and upward; yet you grieve for what you have lost. You know there will be other children and other loving wives, but for now you have the deepest, saddest feelings of desolation.

Element: The element of the chakra is life force. It is not the joyful life force of new beginnings, but life force that is beginning to know sadness and to understand the world. It is life force which, to be itself, must move away and separate from father and mother. Just as the mother bears the child and feels joy at the birth, so she feels loss of the life force that was within her, for now the child must develop by itself.

Sound: The sound of the chakra is that of delicate silver chains being broken. The chains of love bind you to another living being, but these chains are now broken and are falling softly to the ground. The OM chanted here as the mantra of the chakra has a certain harshness about it. This is created by cutting off the silent M before it has faded to stillness to lend a sudden stillness and quiet emptiness to the chant before the OM begins again.

Animal: The animal associated with this chakra is a tiger under control and being used as a beast of burden. To anyone who has taken a cat for a walk on a leash, the thought of being able to ride a tiger brings full realization to this imagery. There is a sadness that this feline beast of the jungle has been brought

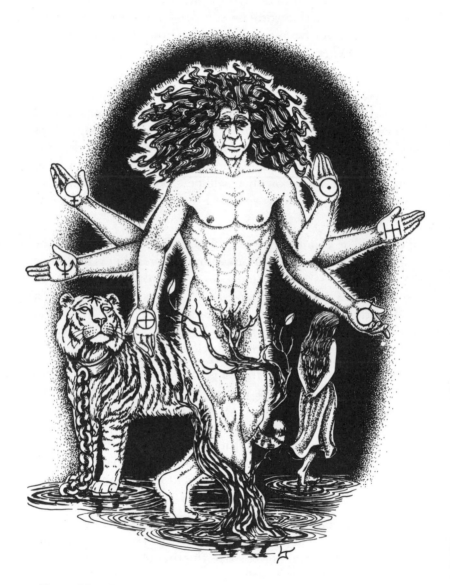

Figure 32.   Shiva.

under control, but simultaneously a knowledge that all savagery must finally be brought under control.

A modern picture of the chakra is that of a man and a woman at last going their separate ways. They have been deeply emotionally involved to such an extent that they were one, but now they must separate and return to the mundane world.

Material: The material of the chakra is the surface of cool water. At first the surface is plain and unrippled. As you get into the chakra, you see that faint images of the world are reflected in the water. The water is stirred by a gentle yet cold psychic breeze that slightly mars the lustrous mirror surface.

Texture: The textural feel of the chakra is that of the finest silk. Silk is light and ethereal, but it is also slightly sensual. When you touch it, you feel uplifted at its wondrous lightness and at the same time are brought into contact with a hint of sensuality.

Smell: The smell of the chakra starts with the smell of new life — the washed-clean baby, either human or animal. It is clean; it has the smell of warmth and life about it. Here the mother has patted it down with some talcum powder. The faint lavender smell of the talc brings to mind the bright purple of the living blossom, along with fading pictures of grandmothers within grandmothers within grandmothers. The line of grandmotherliness stretches back in an infinitude of recurring life that will not be denied, but that also recognizes there is something beyond life which causes this recycling of time.

Taste: The taste of the chakra is water. You are drinking cool spring water, but behind that taste there is a taste of life. If you imagine the taste to be faintly adulterated with that of the sweet redness of watermelon, you can begin to comprehend how the purity of the water — the purity of your spiritual understanding — is being adulterated by things of this world.

God: The god of the chakra is Shiva (figure 32). He is totally white. He glows brilliantly with the inner light of knowledge. He

looks young; he acts young. Yet his eyes reveal that he knows
everything and has seen everything. Slowly he dances the mys-
terious dance of knowledge in a five-beat pattern so that no two
steps are repeated. In his six hands he holds all the six directions
of the world. He gestures to say that he understands, that he is
joyful, and that he will share his joy with you if you only ask for
it. Because he knows everything, in this stage he is the Lord of
Knowledge and Light. In some ways he is the Ultimate Guru
who is your ultimate master.

He brings this illumination to Shakti. When he touches her,
she, too, lights up as a beacon to guide you. Shiva and Shakti
encourage you to impart to the rest of the world the knowledge
you have gained.

Ritual for Illuminating the
Brow Chakra

Before coming to this ritual, the members of the house lightly
paint their faces white or grease their faces and powder them
with talc. Their robes are made of opaque white fabric. They
bring to the ritual a dark red lipstick. They stand in a circle not
touching each other. With eyes closed they intone the O<u>M</u>,
remembering that the silent vibratory <u>M</u> is cut short. Slowly
and carefully they dance in the circle, taking four quick steps
and then one very slow step. After a period they all feel is
appropriate, they stop dancing. They turn to each other and use
the lipstick gently to mark the third eye in red on the brow of
their dyadic partner. Still facing each other, they look deep into
the partner's eyes and smile in recognition. With the right hand
they reach forward and gently scrape away some of the paint or
talc from the left cheek of the partner.

Now they dance as a couple, slowly and sadly, still remembering the physical joy they shared and the spiritual oneness
they so recently abandoned. Gradually the tempo of the dance
picks up. They move into a closer embrace. They are willingly
surrendering the spiritual oneness which they experienced as a

singularity, and are coming back into the world with understanding and comprehension, bringing into their lives the new
illuminated knowledge from their experience. Finally with a
long friendly kiss the ritual ends.

Guided Meditation

Imagine yourself to be a fragmented being. Part of you is now
beyond the Beyond. Another part is in the smoke of a candle
flame. Yet a third part is in the center of a warm friendly bowl of
water. Each part of you has gained new knowledge. Each part of
you very much likes the place where it finds itself. It is as if you
had been on three separate vacations, but you had taken them
all at the same time.

Gradually the three separate parts of your mind bring your
three beings back together. Rise out of the water. Rise above the
candle flame. Come back from the space beyond the Beyond.
Slowly and surely bring these three fragments of your being
toward the center of your brow. Although you do your best to
draw them slowly, as they approach your brow they begin to
move more quickly. Each fragment is eager to recombine with its
fellows. Now you cannot prevent their onward rush. For a
moment you fear a violent collision, but it does not happen;
instead they meld smoothly together and you are one again and
can feel the ground below your buttocks.

Wait now and meditate, opening to what you have
experienced.

ILLUMINATING THE THROAT CHAKRA

The illuminated high which you were on is gently being brought
down. The body that was asleep or in a state of suspended
animation gradually awakens, revitalized, into full invigorating
life. Its physical and spiritual experiences have left it drained of
physical desire, but full of knowledge of its own spirituality. A

little part of the mind remembers the pleasure, and in some ways this clouds the spirituality. The signposts for illuminating the throat chakra are as follows:

Symbol: The moon is waning. It is still almost full size, yet a dark crescent has appeared with its points turned downward. If you gaze carefully at the moon, you can see the very faint outline of this dark shadowy crescent. Though you have almost all its light, you know that the shadow will gradually obscure it, just as you know you will once again be forced into the mundane world.

The petals of the blossoms on your flowering tree are in full flower and abundance. You can easily see sixteen of them. They are beautiful in their newness and freshness. Beneath your admiration of the fullness of their beauty is the knowledge that eventually they will fall and be replaced with older, more knowing petals and flowers.

Color: The color of the chakra is ivory. It is still a lustrous color, but the white purity that you bring with you is tinged with the yellowness of age and earthiness. The body of your being is moving to encase and entrap the perfection of your spirit.

Emotion: The overriding emotion of the chakra is that of gentleness. You are coming from a place where there is no possible conception of evil, no possible conception of hurt or any sort of pain. You believe that by bringing this gentleness into the world, by giving it freely to others, the sweetness and nectar of your love will engender in others the same absolute gentleness that you feel.

Element: The element here is creation. The ultimate life force with which you have melded is the underlying, most powerful, most perfect, and most pure force in the multiverse. Having approached it, you know that it contains awesome power. But you also know that it sits in absolute, silent, clamorous serenity, moving and motionless, with and without desire and all other human emotions. It operates in the world through you. You must use this ultimate force that you have now experienced for creative good in the mundane world.

Sound: The sound of the chakra is that of a flute lightly played, each note being lower than the previous one. The cycle is repeated. The first note is very high and almost inaudible. The last note is low and clearly heard. It represents the downward progression you are making, bringing with you those things that are not of this world to illuminate those around you.

The mantra is HO<u>M</u>. It is sounded progressively as with the notes of the flute, starting high and coming down to lower deeper sounds. In all, eight repetitions of the notes bring you from the high eerie sound down to the low earth sound.

Animal: The animal of the chakra is the white elephant contentedly surrounded by a herd of similar white elephants. This signifies that you will be more content if you are in a group of people who have had training and experiences similar to your own. If you meet someone who has not had the sacred experiences, the encounter will be abrasive. The chakra combines the contentedness and closeness of the family feeling with the slight tinge of roughness that comes from knowing that the world is unable to comprehend your illuminated awareness.

The chakra also shows power and strength from knowledge, for the strength of a herd of white elephants is legendary.

Material: The material of the chakra is ivory. It is a precious, rare substance and is finely carved. When you first obtained this beautiful carving, it appeared to you as lustrous white; but now when you look upon it very carefully, you see it has a tinge of yellow. In some ways the yellow makes it even more beautiful, for it is the yellow of the wisdom of age. In its age and familiarity, the ivory is even more precious to you.

Texture: The texture and feel of the chakra are that of smooth fur. Perhaps it is the underbelly fur that a cat will let you stroke when it's contented and well-fed, when it has nothing to prove and it trusts your good intentions. It is a friend at this moment.

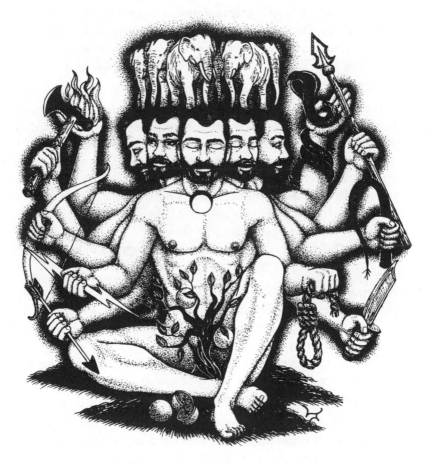

Figure 33.   Shadeshiva.

Its jungle instincts are latent and consciously controlled, for this soft fur is the cat's most vulnerable place. It is soft and warm to the touch, yet in some ways touching it can be dangerous.

Smell: Only those who have smelled the fragrance of real orange blossoms as they waft from the orange grove on the night air can appreciate the subtle hint of beauty that it brings after a long dry day as the dew settles. Most scents that purport to be orange blossom do not catch this hint and subtlety, for they are too cloying and heavy. You know that it will fade, but you know that in the future the sweet oranges will come to fruition and feed your mundane body.

Taste: The taste of the chakra is that of the orange. You taste it first very lightly in pure spring water. Gradually, as you contemplate the chakra, the taste grows stronger and you begin to feel the texture of the fruit in your mouth as well as its taste.

God: The god who illuminates this chakra is Shadeshiva (figure 33). Shiva himself is being overlaid by the things of this world. The throat chakra controls all the senses and limbs of the body. It is a combination of the mind and action, and with his five heads Shadeshiva experiences individualistically the five senses.

In each hand he holds weapons. These remind you that the place you are about to enter contains pain and hurt and war— many negative things. He also holds a beautiful cobra, one you much admire but can never quite trust. The noose is there to symbolize death. His other hands indicate the very positive illuminated emotions you have brought with you down into this chakra—goodness, courage to try again, and firmness—for no matter what the world throws at you now, you have glimpsed the ultimate truth. The illuminated Shadeshiva causes the goddess of the chakra, Shakini, also to be illuminated. She, too, strives for goodness and courage, and gives these qualities to her children.

Ritual for Illuminating the
Throat Chakra

The members of the house are dressed in opaque robes of pale beige. They bring to the ritual area any weapons they may have. A small fire is lighted at the center of the area. This is often a fire of alcohol burning on a sand base. The flame is almost invisible. Yet its heat can be felt and if you look carefully you can see its clear blueness. Members of the house form no particular pattern or grouping. They wander around showing one another the weapons they carry. The edges of the sword or a knife are tested. Small pieces of paper may be cut up or stabbed. The mantra HO<u>M</u> is started. At first only the yogins sing rather than chant it. Then as the pitch is lowered, the yogis join in, and after eight repetitions the final chant is done in a deep low voice by the yogis. On the next repetition of the mantra, the weapons are laid down in a circle. The members form a circle within the circle of weapons, facing outward into the world with the flame of inspiration behind them. Now they back toward the flame. They place their arms around each other's waist to form a locked tight circle. While they are tightly arranged thus, they begin to step sideways rapidly in a clockwise direction. This requires that everyone step in unison and the mantra is used to set the step frequency. Some practice is required to make this locked rotating arrangement work; and even after practice the occasional stumble will occur. Anyone who stumbles is helped up and firmly re-melded into the unity of the locked circle.

After a further eight mantric chants, the rotation is slowed and stopped. The members strain outward as if trying to get away from the circle. Then they fall back in on themselves so they lean backward with heads held back over the alcohol flame. This pulsating motion is also repeated eight times. When it is complete, the circle is broken and all pat and caress one another, lightly kissing male and female alike, content in the knowledge of shared experience and mutual support and strength.

Guided Meditation

Come with me to a past time of battle, tribe against tribe, person against person. You can see their pain and you can see their futile battles. It is a dark and somber scene. You can smell blood. But also you can smell the sweet perfume you have brought with you. You are a being of light. As you come into the scene, all people stop fighting and gaze on you. You see a person with a broken limb. You use the haft of a battle axe as a splint and you use someone else's dagger to cut vines to bind the splint to the broken limb. After it is bound, you caress it with your hand and it is healed. Those around you come to you to plead for sustenance. Instead of giving them things of this earth, you reach to touch their minds with your illuminated knowledge. As you touch their minds, they stop fighting and begin to cultivate the earth with their weapons. Some swords are turned into plowshares.

As you watch, new life comes from the ground. You know you have changed the spirit of the people, and the spirit of the people has changed their minds, and their minds have changed the actions of their bodies. You watch in wonder as groves of trees grow on the plains. You watch in wonder as other people come and see the change wrought by your illuminated presence. Sit and watch now as the change spreads outward, as whole nations lay down their weapons simply because an illuminated one has made its presence felt.

Come back now slowly and reluctantly to the real world in which you live, resolved to help others by giving them some of your inner light, not by giving them mundane goods and services.

ILLUMINATING THE HEART CHAKRA

In this mode of illumination, the heart chakra is one of altruistic love. The word "love" is extremely difficult to define, for "love" means something different to each person. Perhaps this is the love of a father for his children, or the love of a mother for her children. There is no sexual connotation involved. It is just the hope that the children will live to their full potential and will come to full perfect maturity. The animal instincts within each of them are to be accepted by the parents and the child is to be trained in understanding so that he or she can accept his or her instincts, understand them, and perhaps use them so that each will attain full potential. The signposts for illuminating the heart chakra are as follows:

Symbol: The symbol for the chakra is the lotus and its petals. Here you see that as you come down into the world, four of the petals have already been lost, for coming into the world has meant some loss, and some coarsening of your finer feelings. Another symbol is hidden in the chakra—the undying flame of pure love. Pure and clear is this flame, yet it burns with a yellow tinge for it is a flame of this world. If allowed out of control, it can consume everything in its path. The mother or father seeing a child threatened will exhibit this flame of passionate protection and the flame will burn, and if necessary destroy, the attacker.

Color: The color of the chakra is a smoky blue. In India after the dry season, the distant clouds of the monsoon may disturb the purity of the blue sky; but they are welcome, for the deep smoky blueness of their underside denotes that the rain god has not forgotten you and will shortly come to nurture his children. Thus the blue is the blueness of the underside of a heavy rain cloud in a bright blue sky. It is not a clear blue, for it has gray in it, but it is a friendly nurturing color foretelling good things— not in any way a cold blue.

Emotion: The emotion of the chakra is languor. The listlessness of waiting for something to happen is predominant here. In some ways, your emotions have been used up by your almost traumatic climb up through the chakras and your confrontation with your mirrored oneness in the ultimate experience. What more can happen to you? Why should you do anything? For whatever you do, what will be will be. This languor is mixed with regret that you are back in the world and must now look after the children you love. You know that very soon you must rouse yourself and go out and begin to make things happen again.

Element: The element of air rules this chakra. It is the air that you see expelled with the breath. As the life force comes into a living creature, so that creature begins to inhale and exhale the vital air it needs for life. This chakra contains the exhaled air. Perhaps it is the carbon dioxide that is turned into oxygen by green and living things or the carbon dioxide that a living being expels that has been made from the oxygen of the air. Whatever its chemical constituents, still it is vital air that has been used once and was changed by its contact with a living being.

Sound: In the distance you can hear the sound of bells. They are summoning you back into the world, where you are supposed to join with masses of other people and perform rituals under the control of those who ring the bells. At present they are muffled and very distant, but you know that soon they will become louder and more insistent. Whether or not you join in the rituals of others you know that your own consciousness—the "Me" that is within you—will cause your body to enact rituals of eating, working, loving, and sleeping. You will enjoy some of these rituals, and you promise yourself that you will rise above them. You know that in some ways it is an empty promise; for in the great cycle of your life there are small cycles that are ever repetitive, and soon you will be caught up in the smallness of some of those cycles. You realize as you listen to the power of the muffled bells that inevitably there is a great cycle within which you perform your small part.

The mantra is softly repetitive and sounds like bells in the distance. It is often performed without opening the teeth so that it always has a muffled cadence. It is YA<u>M</u>. It should be repeated within the mind as often as is necessary to bring the muffled bells and their significance into your awareness.

Animal: The black antelope is the animal of this chakra. It is under the control of a rider who rides it comparatively lightly, for the antelope is a willing steed. It is black—black as midnight. Within its ultimate blackness there is every color. Since it is so perfectly black, every single color must be balanced within it; when you enter the blackness of its color, you will go through it and see the individual separated colors in brilliant array. The antelope is a strong swift animal. It will carry you back swiftly into your workplace. It is under control, not bounding freely; but it is happy in its control for it knows you will release it to run free as soon as you have ridden it a little. The antelope's life cannot always be the pure pleasure of running free and uninhibited. Sometimes it must be willing to act as a steed so it can understand more fully the pleasures inherent in freedom.

Material: The material of the chakra is a red ruby that glows with a beautiful inner light even when it is set in a dark place. The ruby contains the knowledge you have gained in your travels through the chakras. It serves to remind you that you have within a priceless jewel that will illuminate you in the darkest moments of your despair. It can be gazed upon and admired by others who have traveled paths similar to yours—but cannot be seen by those with little or no awareness. When others gaze on your ruby of knowledge, your own personal jewel, they take nothing from you; for the jewel glows whether or not anyone looks at it. If they come to berate you and criticize and denigrate your ruby, you must put it out of sight. You must hide it within your heart chakra and not let them see it. For the ruby can in fact be shattered by emotions of jealousy, envy, resentment, and self-doubt. If dulled, the ruby can be instantly rekindled with the love and illumination that you gain from your upward path and from the love you bear your children.

Texture: The texture and feel of the chakra is that of a strongly beating heart. The muscles work well to pump blood strongly through your body. As the muscles work, the skin of your chest is pressed outward and then relaxed. Imagine the feeling you get from the inside of your skin as it is pressed outward when you clench and unclench. It is a tightening feeling, but pleasurable and reassuring, for it signifies that all is well. The heart is working properly and your skin feels healthy and flexible. Getting inside yourself and experiencing this feeling are sure ways of getting into tune with the chakra when it is entered from above.

Smell: The scent of the chakra is that of a deep velvet red rose. It is the scent of altruistic love unspoiled by any lustful or sexual desire. There is hope here that the person receiving the rose will recognize it as a symbol of pure unselfish love. The scent is deep and strong. It makes your whole being vibrate with the same vibration that you felt when you repeated the mantra.

Taste: The taste of the chakra can be compared to that of a ripe pineapple. It is a full taste without bitterness. Once experienced, it can never be forgotten. The pineapple gives up its sweetness and its fruit so that future generations of pineapples are protected and can grow.

God: The god of this chakra is Isha, who glows with inner self-confidence and love (figure 34 on page 228). If you allow it, he will love you and the whole world. Yet he has a somewhat repulsive countenance. He looks dangerous. He has three eyes. You notice that his third eye is somewhat closed. He is stationary and fixed, but in his symbology lies tremendous strength of purpose. Nothing will change him. He will remain fixed forever, just as parental love never changes. Even when a child disappoints his or her parent, still the good parent loves the child. Thus it is with Isha. The luster of his love illuminates the chakra. His light is white but tinged with the redness of ruby, so that overall it appears as a light orange.

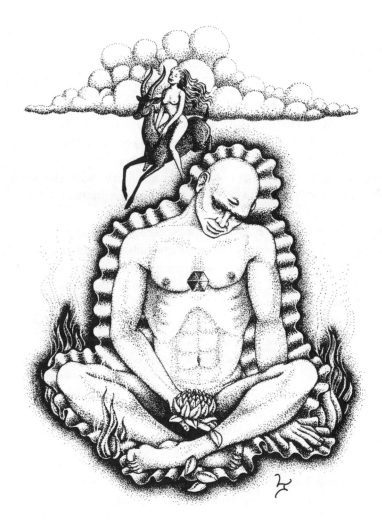

Figure 34.   Isha.

Ritual for Illuminating the
Heart Chakra

The members of the house come into the exercise area wearing clothing which is most appropriate for children. Each carries a lighted black candle. They put their candles in a circle at the center of the exercise area. They hug one another and they kiss and cuddle. Some pretend to be hurt, and get other members to comfort them. They are totally childish in their behavior. One may throw a tantrum, another may squeal. All this childish behavior is carried on with much hugging, kissing on the forehead and cheek, and soft caressing. After some minutes of this behavior, one of the members starts the mantra YA<u>M</u> at a very low pitch, in a voice that sounds distant and soft. Everyone listens. Soon they begin to join in until all are sounding the mantra. As they sound it, they remove their childish clothes, revealing the adult bodies underneath. Yet still they hug and kiss one another, not on the mouth but on the cheek and the forehead. They do everything they can to express their altruistic love of one another. Typically they massage one another with rose-scented oil. They comb one another's hair, cut one another's nails, and groom one another. Any area of skin that is rough, or any injury, is carefully attended to. Every member of the house pays particular attention to the hurt. This activity continues until all grow tired and in dyadic pairs they leave to continue their quiet embraces and fall asleep in one another's arms.

Guided Meditation

Come into meditation with me in a completely relaxed and sexually fulfilled condition. You are going to meditate in a way that breaks the rules of meditation. You will meditate cuddled together with your dyadic partner. It is important that you both be very comfortable and that you are able to retain this position for the length of the meditation. One good way to do this is to lie in bed together with your heads facing north. You are comfortable, held in the arms of one you absolutely trust. You know that if anything comes in that might remotely harm you, your partner will rise up and protect you from it, burning away any possible threat to you in the fire of loving protection.

Imagine now that you are deep inside a red ruby. Its outer surface is so hard that it will protect you against everything. In here there is a pure white light that appears red to those outside because it is colored by the ruby itself. As you look through the ruby at the world, you don't see its negative aspects, for every scene you view has a rosy hue added to it by the ruby's color. You are in here. You are protected. The world is a good place to be in.

Look now at the white light. It is the light of your own secret knowledge. You find you can make the light burn more brightly or more dimly. You turn it down until it is almost off. You don't like that—so gradually, ever so slowly, you increase its brilliance. As you increase the brilliance of the light, you remember with love the help your partner gives you toward attaining your goal of oneness and knowledge.

Now the light is beginning to hurt your eyes. You cannot really look at it, and you leave it at this brilliance, for it is all the knowledge and light that you can grasp at your present stage of awareness. You are content in the knowledge that with the loving help of your companion, you will be able to increase the strength of the light in the future. Now tend your light in the safety at the center of the jewel of your knowledge. Be quiet now. Sleep in loving protection.

ILLUMINATING THE NAVEL CHAKRA

As you descend into the navel chakra, you know you are again approaching the deep dark emotional upheaval that is inherent in your sensual being and which is governed by the reptilian part of the brain outside the control of the spirit. You are angry that your body is once again asserting its needs, but your earlier understanding of your needs lends you the strength to venture down into the lower chakras. The signposts for illuminating the navel chakra are as follows:

Symbol: The swastika symbol of eternal good fortune rules this chakra. You know that you are very lucky to have had the experiences given to you. Your good fortune will come again, so you are happy that you are entering this chakra—yet the happiness is mixed with annoyance that you must follow a downward path. The petals of your lotus, or your flowering tree (whichever you prefer), are tinged with the golden colors of autumn. They are about to fall as the tree loses the fresh green of early summer. But you know that after the autumn and after the winter it (and you, yourself) will be reborn. There is a sadness but a completion in the color of the petals.

Color: The blue-gray of the thunderclouds has left you. Now fire burns the fallen branches. This is a sacred fire caused by lightning. Its smoke is white. The symbology of the chakra combines the white smoke with the light blue of the autumn sky.

Emotion: The emotion of the chakra is laziness. You know you should be doing something, you know you should be moving, but you are too lazy to do it. In some ways this is a negative emotion, lacking spirit and motivation. There are things you ought to be doing, but you are simply too lazy—to willfully self-indulgent—to get up and do them. Inside, you are a little disgusted with yourself for being so lazy, but this is not really disgust; it is just a certain old sadness that you—who have been such a high-spirited motivated being—have fallen prey to this self-indulgent mood.

Element: The element of the chakra is the mundane fire. The breath of life has made everything grow in wild disarray and abandon. All your thoughts have strayed and become entangled and ensnared in one another. The purifying fire is used to transform the worthless tangled underbrush into good new nutrients. You must put from your mind things that would hinder a clear

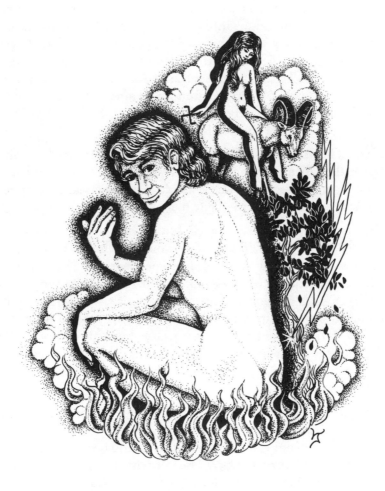

Figure 35. Rudra.

perception of your path. You must put aside such mundane things as feeling disgust or repulsion at the behavior which you know you will soon indulge in again. Your inner fire and determination must be rekindled. This determination is tempered by actions to come. You know that shortly you will be letting the baser instincts have full rein and you must be determined that they shall have full rein, that you will abandon yourself to the path on which you find yourself. Now you are in control. You can enjoy this control, though you know that the reins will soon again be loosed.

Sound: The sound of the chakra is the beat of thunder. It is always in the background. It is very softly heard, but it is growing more intense and more insistent. The thunder approaches. It is not threatening, but it is very real. For now, your gathering excitement is firmly reined in and held in check. Yet even though it is reined in, you feel a certain dryness in the throat and a heightening awareness of what the future holds.

The mantra of the chakra is RA<u>M</u>, but it is pronounced more as ra<u>m</u> with a very short, silent <u>M</u>. It starts very softly and builds slowly, reminding you of approaching thunder and of the rampant nature of the ram.

Animal: The animal of the chakra is the ram. In heat it is violent, berserk, and a representation of the reproductive force of nature. Here, however, the ram is kept in control by a rider. The rider represents your mind, and behind the rider is your spirit. The ram is there. It is under control. There is a feeling of natural underlying latent reproductive force.

Material: The material of the chakra is soft red gold. The gold is brought from the furnace and may be molded to any shape. It is up to your desire—do you want a beautiful shape, a savage shape, or just a meaningless shape? The gold is your toy. No matter what you do to it or how you handle it, its lustrous light will not tarnish. This is the secret—for (provided you retain your inner light and direction) short of destroying the gold, nothing you do will cause it to lose its inner glow.

Texture: The texture and feel of the chakra is that of soft leather. The leather is strong and can protect you. It can be formed into gloves to protect your hands from heat and damage. Yet it is also soft and sensual, showing that sensuality is not necessarily a sign of weakness. Instead it can be a sign of strength for those who can understand, comprehend, and come to terms with it.

Smell: One of the smells perhaps most easily brought to mind for this chakra is that of leaves being burned on a sunny autumn afternoon. The smell is sweet, yet its perfume is of the woods, free of artifice. It reminds you that because of the fire, nutrients will be produced to fertilize the soil so that new and stronger growth will be produced in the future. It is both a childhood smell and an adult smell, for if the leaves are allowed to lie they will mold. Children can gather them up; it is the adults who apply the flame of understanding and spread the new ashes where they will do the most good.

Taste: The taste of the chakra is dark black rum. The rum has been cured in casks that have had their insides burned to form charcoal. The blackness and the darkness of the sugarcane syrup come through to you.

God: The god of the chakra is Rudra (figure 35 on page 232). At first sight he appears gray-blue; but a closer look reveals he is covered in ashes, and under the ashes his skin is actually aflame and is red. He symbolizes both the fire of inspiration and the red of base desires, all covered in the white ash caused by a passionate understanding. The desire, the inspiration, and the illumination are all hidden from your sight by the gray-white ash. He fearlessly faces the future, and indicates that you, too, should fearlessly come with him along the spiral path.

Ritual for Illuminating the
Navel Chakra

Members enter the exercise area with the genitalia totally covered and confined in heavy gray fabric. In Western houses the breasts of the yogins are also covered in the same fabric. A very faint gray mark is made at the position of the third eye. Each member brings in a gift of food that he or she knows the dyadic partner likes. This can be candy, a piece of meat, anything that is a particular favorite of the partner. Each dyadic couple stands back to back hugging the gift to their chests. All begin the mantric chant in eight repetitions. The chant becomes quite insistent. The couples turn to face in the same direction so their shoulders lean against each other. They show each other the tidbit they are carrying and chant another set of the mantra.

Now they turn to face one another. With the right hand, they reach down to grasp the cloth over each other's yoni and lingam. With the left hand they offer the tidbits. Another mantric chant ram is started. As the chant progresses, the food is brought closer to the partner's lips and the grip on the lingam and the yoni becomes more firm and insistent. Then at the end of the chant, they release their sexual grasp and feed the partner the tidbit. They gently embrace, kissing quite demurely on the cheeks. They retire to their rooms to fulfill their ritual copulation requirements.

Navel Chakra Illumination—
Guided Meditation

You are watching a tiny leaf smoldering away. Every so often it flames brightly. A child comes and adds more leaves to the flame. As the leaves catch fire, the child grows up and becomes the personification of your most perfect lover. You move toward the lover but the fire is between you. Smoke rises and obscures the scene. The fire burns down and you advance toward your lover, but your lover adds more leaves and you must retreat. The ash from the fire covers your lover's skin. Gradually your passionate desire dies away and you, too, begin to gather leaves and burn them on the fire, knowing that when this task is complete, you will be able to make love slowly, surely, completely.

Watch yourself as you gather the leaves. You know that when all the leaves are gathered your time will come. At first you work quickly and you miss many leaves, but you know that every leaf must be gathered away before you can attain fulfillment.

ILLUMINATING THE PELVIC CHAKRA

Now you are beginning once again to enter fully into the reptilian part of the brain—but you are bringing the illumination of your previous upward journey. When you cry for that which is lost, it is as if you are weeping for your own innocent youth. The signposts for illuminating the pelvic chakra are as follows:

Symbol: The symbol of the chakra is six tear-like petals. These are the slightly salt tears that you shed because you know you must give up the spiritual side of your life and come back down into the lusty emotions of the world. In some ways the tears are crocodile tears, because you know you will enjoy the pleasures of the near future.

Color: The color of the chakra is blueness that you brought with you. The blue of the sky is being overshadowed by the greenish-yellow of your emotions. Your purity is being tested, and there are very faint hints of yellow, as if the sun is gently setting on your illuminated knowledge. You should have no fear, for you will not forget the illumination you have received. Instead, you remember that you are seeking more illumination. You change the yellow from a negative greenish tinge to pure golden streaks of hope.

Emotion: The emotions of the chakra combine a wish to remain above and outside the turmoil of the world with the knowledge that only through the fire of that turmoil can you receive future blessings. Without experiencing black, you cannot fully comprehend the beauty of white.

Element: As the fire burns, it can produce from its vapors pure distilled water. The fire can burn you if you venture into it, yet its heat and purifying spirit produce water essential to life.

Sound: The sound of the chakra is a sea calming down. It represents emotion. You know that the sea can be stirred up by your own emotions and become terrible and violent again. For now the sea is calm. Long swells break gently on the beach. The mantra VA<u>M</u> is pronounced with exaggerated slowness and steadiness and smooth repetitiveness. It is the sea, ever present, ever moving, but at present content with its inner power.

Animal: The animal of the chakra is the sleeping crocodile. The crocodile has eaten, and everything in its world is in repose. It has nothing to fear. If it is suddenly awakened, it can use its tremendous power; but it is content. It is resting as you are resting. Though it is of this world, it is dreaming its dream of higher things.

Material: The material of the chakra is a single grain of salt. You have no lust; you have no need to gorge yourself on food; all your senses have been taken care of. But because you are awake and aware with all your senses finely tuned, the taste of one single grain of salt is enough to symbolize all the salt and sensuality in the world.

Texture: The texture of the chakra is already in your imagination. Reach down and feel the outside of your calf. The skin is tight and smooth. Now as you gently stroke it, imagine you are feeling it not from the outside but from the inside. The texture of the skin from the inside of your body is the texture you need to understand for comprehension of the chakra.

Smell: It is cold and you are snuggled down in bed. A stray air current in the house brings to your nose the smell of bread toasting, and you know that someone in the house is up and about. Somewhere, too, you detect an overlying odor of fabric being ironed. The smell of ironed hot cotton is present with the smell of freshly made toast.

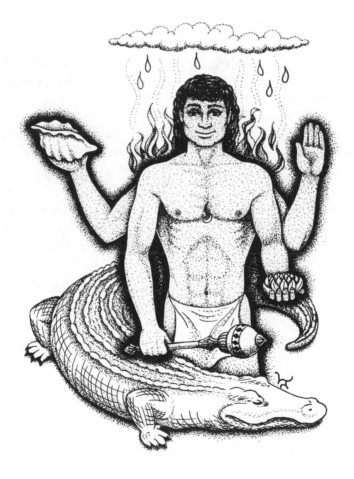

Figure 36.   Vishnu.

Taste: Just as you are stirring and thinking about returning to the world in which you live, someone brings you a delicious cup of morning coffee or tea. The taste is the way you conceive it will taste when you drink it. It is not the actual taste of the tea or coffee; it is the thought of the taste that you anticipate it will have when you actually drink it.

God: The god of the chakra is Vishnu (figure 36). In many ways he is the most romantic love god of the Hindu pantheon. His blue skin shows how aware and spiritual he is. His clothing of light yellow shows that even though he is spiritual, he understands the emotions of the world. To satisfy his lady he will make love; but he would prefer only to bring her jewels and flowers and tenderly look after her and grant her every wish. He is ever-faithful, ever-present; he never puts any pressure whatsoever on those around him. He is reliable, restrained, and relaxing.

On Vishnu's chest is a curl that may be taken for fire. It is part of the spiral of spirituality and development. He has four arms. In his hands he holds a conch to summon other gods to his help if he needs them, and a mace to symbolize the power he can wield in this world if he wishes to. The mace is not raised upward. It is resting. He also carries the ever-present flower that he is about to give his lady. This is always a lotus bloom, for in giving the lotus, he hopes the lady will follow him along the path of enlightenment.

Ritual for Illuminating the Pelvic Chakra

This ritual is the great Maithuna ritual where affection, desire, and sexual activity are restrained by the power of the mind so no orgasm occurs and no lust is displayed. The yogis come to the exercise room wearing a light blue dusting of powder on their faces and upper bodies. Some will have Vishnu's symbol of the curl or flame drawn on their chest, and may carry a lotus. The yogins come with a dusting of light yellow powder or wearing

light yellow robes. They greet one another reverently with a kiss
of hands and fingertips, and perhaps stroking of cheeks or hair.
They form a circle holding hands as couples. One couple does
not hold the hands of the next couple, for each couple is deeply
in love in a romantic way. Each yogi lays a flower at the feet of
his yogin. The yogin does not pick up the flower in the early
part of the ceremony. Quietly they chant the mantra until
everyone is totally fed up with it—far longer than would normally be expected, probably eight minutes in all.

While they chant, the partners gradually turn toward each
other and hold each other in a formal Western dance position,
where the bodies are kept separate. The yogi's right hand rests
on the yogin's waist and her left forearm lies lightly on his right
shoulder. His left hand and her right hand are joined.

When the chant finishes, the yogis pick up the flowers and
offer them again to the yogins. The yogins take them and feel
obligated to give something back—yet they have nothing to
offer except themselves. They approach the yogis more closely
and begin to cuddle. The yogi responds to the caress of the
yogin. She lies on her back and pulls him down to her. He lies
on his side. After more cuddling and kissing, she introduces the
lingam into the yoni, while he remains on his side. As before,
they touch each other except in the area of the lingam and yoni,
though they can make sexual movements with contractions of
the lingam and the yoni. The yogin can try to bring the yogi to
orgasm, but if they get too close, they must back off; for the
whole point of the ritual is that neither partner has an orgasm. It
is especially important that the yogi who portrays Vishnu does
not have an orgasm.

After 32 minutes of this play, the partners rise again to
their feet and repeat their dance-type embrace and their chant.
Often the yogin will place a flower in her hair and one in the
hair of the yogi, but anyone who loses control does not get a
flower.

Guided Meditation

Come with me now out into the calm waves of the Pacific Ocean. You have found a beautiful coral atoll. It is the typical Pacific paradise with waving palm trees, gentle breezes, and a warm sea gently lapping on the beach. You walk out of the green shade of the palm trees. The sun is warm on your naked skin, and the sand is warm and firm under your feet. On the other side of the island waits the lover who lives with you. You are content.

As you look, you see a passenger liner steaming across the horizon. Smoke comes from its funnels. You imagine you hear music and see thousands of people on board. Some weeks ago you prepared a beacon fire; but you have grown so content that now you look at the collected wood and wonder whether you should light it. Will you light the beacon or not? If you don't light it, will you tell your lover about the ship? You lie down in the warm sun at the edge of the water and meditate on your decision.

As the liner sails away, the world is leaving you. You are alone and content in your tropical paradise. Presently you feel the steps of your lover approaching. Meditate on the action you will take. Watch yourself get up and . . .

Come back now from your meditation with the full feeling of the pelvic chakra, as you leave it to come farther down into the world in the base chakra.

ILLUMINATING THE BASE CHAKRA

The base chakra symbolizes the world. You enter it from above only with reluctance. You have experienced every sensual pleasure and passion, and you are fed up with the world. Though you long to transcend it, you know you must re-enter it; more-over, you must tell others of your experiences to compensate the gods for what you have learned. Few can understand you, few will listen, but teach you must, and to teach you must re-enter the world. You are old in wisdom and the world is full of folly. You would much prefer to wrap your arms around yourself, hug the knowledge to yourself, and live a hermit-like existence, but that is not the Tantric way. The Tantric path makes you live in the world, experiencing its passions and pain. You must overcome them. The signposts for illuminating the base chakra are as follows:

Symbol: The symbol of the chakra is the four remaining petals on your flowering tree or on the dying lotus. Only the four petals remain. They are symmetrically arranged to point in the four directions of the mundane world. The petals are old and stained with the dried blood of the world. The feeling is, "Do I want to go through all that again?" even while you know the answer is "Yes." The petals tell you that you should choose one direction, go into the world, and pursue it until you can come back up through this chakra again on your way toward greater awareness. The blood is your blood, spilled perhaps in your effort to shape the world to your will or simply working in the world. The blood is dried because (you hope) you will have to spill no more.

Color: The color of the chakra is the color of autumn in a deciduous forest. The leaves are deep red and brown. You are surrounded by the death of the old, which you know will result next year in birth of the new. From death life is reborn; but you cannot help being sad for the trees that have lost their vivid green foliage. In some ways the color is very attractive. Every year thousands of people go out to look at the colors of the fall foliage. This is the color you are seeing.

Emotion: The emotion of the chakra is contentment after fulfillment. You have had a fight with a loved one and have reconciled. You have made love. Perhaps you have also gone to the bathroom and had a very satisfactory bowel movement. You are empty; your passions—both verbal and sexual—are spent. You would like to crawl back under your blanket and spend the next week in bed. But you have work to do.

Element: The element of the chakra is good fertile earth. Perhaps a farmer understands and appreciates this more than a city dweller does. The earth is black, damp, and crumbly. It is warm and granular. It is rich; it smells of future life.

Sound: The sound is distant drums beating with the pulse of the world in a regular pattern and rhythm. You can imagine people dancing and being turned on by the drums. Yet they are not getting nearer; you must go to them if you want to hear them more clearly.

The mantra is LAM. The L is like a beat on a drum, rounded and full. It is not a loud mantra; instead it is a soft calling mantra, calling you into the world.

Animal: The animal of the chakra is a quiet powerful working elephant. The elephant is fully under control, doing heavy labor, lifting logs and placing them in a neat stack. The only sound is the dull plod of the elephant's feet, the dull thump as the log goes down. It is an age-old working scene. The dead trees will be used to build houses. The elephant's rider instructs by pressure from his knees. The two minds have perfect understanding.

Material: The material of the chakra is sandstone. It is red because it has a high iron content. In fact there are streaks in it where water has run over it. This is not a tiny piece of sandstone, but a large cliff. It has been there since the world was young and will gradually wear away, for it is a soft comfortable rock with rounded surfaces, free of sharp edges that would cut you.

Texture: The feel is that of the good earth. An easy way to experience it is to dip your fingers into a package of soft brown sugar and feel the granularity, softness, and warmth of it.

Smell: The smell of the chakra is that of the harvest, scenting the air first when the hay is mowed and again when the corn is cut.

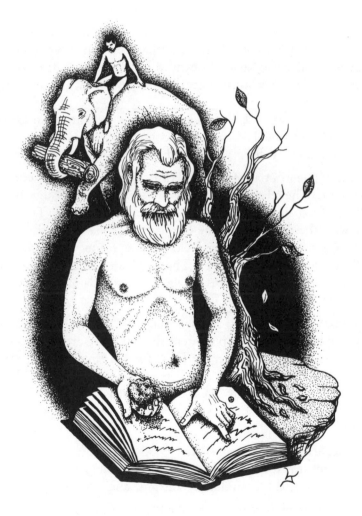

Figure 37.   Brahma.

There may be a tinge of wood smoke in the air as the smell changes from summer hay to the burning stubble of autumn.

Taste: The taste is of the earth, perhaps resembling a carrot that has been lightly cooked. The taste contains all the earthy goodness that nature provides. It is sweet and good, with a certain texture. It reawakens your taste buds to the stronger tastes of the earth.

God: The god of the chakra is Brahma (figure 37). The wise knowledgeable teacher is the aspect of Shiva that resides in this chakra. Many will not listen to him. Many are so taken up with the pleasures and sensuality of the earth that they cannot be bothered with him. Yet he continues to teach with great kindness and understanding the ones who come to him. He never raises his voice, nor does he use the whip. Instead, he is full of patient teaching so that those around get a glimpse of his spirituality. He uses hundreds of symbols and stories in teaching his wisdom to worldly people.

Ritual for Illuminating the Base Chakra

This ritual is done in the morning before anyone leaves the house for work. All meet together in the exercise room. While they huddle as closely and as tightly together as they can, either standing or lying on the floor, they gently sound the mantra LA<u>M</u> with its insistent drumming L. They exchange many caresses and press foreheads together. All know they must soon leave the security, friendship, and understanding of the group and go out into the world. When the mantra is finished, they regretfully stop the kissing and cuddling and forehead touching. They stand facing outward with their backs to each other and holding each other tightly around the waist, their arms behind them. They lean backward toward one another then walk slowly apart, their arms pulled from around one another's waists. They all dress slowly in their outdoor working clothes and leave the house.

If they are full-time residents, working only within the house, still they must leave the house and do some mundane task, such as shopping. This would be a good time to teach if that is what you do.

Guided Meditation

Come with me now. You are in a forest. A pleasant path runs beside a tinkling stream. In the distance you hear music with an insistent drumbeat in it. It is autumn. The leaves have all turned a beautiful reddish brown. Many have already fallen, and as you walk along the path some of them rustle under your tread. You are drawn toward the music, yet it is pleasant here in the forest. The path wends its way down hill. As you come down, in the distance you see the trees are still green and fresh as if it is still springtime below. Now above the music you hear the voices of young people. The path comes to a wall surrounding your part of the forest. The wall is old and gray and covered with lichen.

You see a gate in the wall. At first you are reluctant to open it, but eventually the music calls you on and you open the gate. You find yourself in a room that you have built for yourself. Here you find books and tools of your trade. By the glow that comes from them, you can tell they are magical. You take with you what you know you will need when you get to the place of the music. With some reluctance, but now with more confidence, you leave your room and re-enter the world.

As you come back from your meditation and find yourself in your own place, pay special attention to the way your room is furnished and consider which of the magical tools or books to take with you. The furnishings give you a clue to your heritage, and the tools reveal what your natural mission in the world will be.

CHAPTER
TEN

Understanding Your
Spiral Dance

IT IS APPARENT that early humans tried to make bargains with their deities via the path of sacrifice. They were no strangers to the hardships of life; and the thought of sacrifice as something a god would appreciate was easy to understand. The concept of human sacrifice was born when the idea was implanted that the spirit of the victim who went willingly to the sacrifice would be the deity's companion and could intercede to ask for favors on behalf of the tribe. The sacrifice to a goddess would be the most handsome young man and the sacrifice to a god the most beautiful maiden. To a deity of another aspect (the god of the herd of goats, for instance) it was more appropriate to sacrifice the most perfect goat or ram, and to a corn god, the most perfect ears of corn. All deities appreciated food, since they were believed to exist on the spiritual part of it—the early manna from earth. Since only the spirit went onward and upward, after the appropriate ceremony the tribe could eat the offering. Early hunters made promises to the deity before going on the hunt, dedicating the spirit of the animal they killed to the Great Spirit of that animal.

Soon it became apparent that the more spirits sacrificed, the better was the chance the deity would listen to requests and be pleased with the attention it got. This is the earliest form of the god-bargain: "I am doing this for you; therefore when I ask you to do something, you should do it for me." At this stage, religion was active and sacrificial. As people moved into cities and away from the influences of the land and of nature, so religion became more of the mind; and worship and prayer were offered to the god in lieu of sacrifices. Even now it is easy to fall back into the old ways and make promises like, "God! If I get out of this I'll go to church for six months!"

The next stage of religious development is the coalescing of multiple anthropomorphic deities into a single anthropomorphic deity that also has some ideomorphic or transcendent qualities. Even though the religion still has its ritualistic behavior, it has become passive, with only a handful of priests and cult figures officiating and taking active part in the new form of godbargain: "All these people will worship and praise you and in return you will do me many favors," with "All these people will worship and praise," replacing ideomorphically the earlier sacrifice.

From this point on, in most cases the emphasis on the transcendent part of the deity is diminished. The particular cult figure becomes more and more an idol and the vast mass of people are encouraged to be idolators; for all the cult leaders want is that the energy contained in the people's prayers and worship shall be directed to the cult's favorite idol.

You can see this change clearly in the Old Testament. Early sacrifice is replaced with worship. Abraham—once he is willing to sacrifice his son—is told that it is no longer necessary. The Golden Calf is cast down. Yet Jehovah remains throughout because the early all-powerful volcano god, transformed first to a barley god and then to a father figure, was too well entrenched in Jewish consciousness to be replaced. The anthropomorphic sacrificial deity has been replaced with the ideomorphic worship deity.

In Hinduism both religious ideas are retained; the old sacrificial part remains, and the worship-and-prayer part is grafted onto it. In historical fact we know that the Eastern Valley people whose culture came to a height in the period immediately after

3,000 BCE were the protean people of a sacrificial religion and the invading Aryans brought with them their ideomorphic religion. Instead of the sacrificial religion being bloodily suppressed in attempts to extinguish it, the two religions were brought together and made one whole. Not only that, but deity names from various subgroups were brought in to fill appropriate slots in the pantheon, so that everyone could worship or sacrifice (or combine worship and sacrifice) to whatever deity was comfortable and necessary to their wholeness and physical well-being. "We priests understand, of course, that these are all aspects of our own supreme deities, Shakti and Shiva; so we'll let the people go on worshipping the deities they like."

CREATION

If you look at very early creation myths, you find that things are created from the materials of the earth. "Mud is taken and formed into the shape of man and woman and life is breathed into them," says the Popul Vuh. As the world grew older, so a more philosophical view of creation came into vogue and emphasis was placed on creation from a divine First Source. This creation, too, can be of the old nature or earth-first, which is then populated, or of the spirit-first, which then creates the world. If you look at the symbology of Tantra, you can see that both natural and divine creations are accommodated. A child taking earth, adding water, and baking it, can create an idol. A philosophy student can imagine that all that is created flows from a divine source. Figure 38 on page 250 shows this. The creation from nature is shown on the left. From the womb of the Great Mother, the earth is created. On the earth water is formed and on the water fire flickers. From the fire air rises and from all this the world is created. Soon after that life comes into the world. The spirit of life, when it gains awareness, creates a

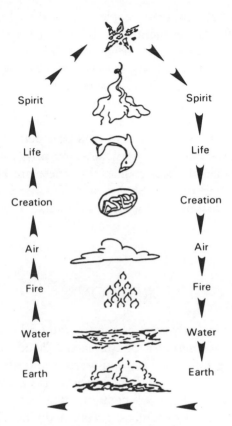

Figure 38.   Creation from above and below.

pantheon of gods and goddesses. Everything is created from the original Great Mother. The chakras are ascended and activated.

Conversely, in the right side of the figure you see the divine-creation concept. God creates the spirit, which creates life. Life then creates a world in which to live and then puts into the world the elements of the world: first air to breathe, then fire, then water; and from the water the earth arises. The chakras are descended and illuminated.

Figure 38 is really a continuous loop, for once earth is created, you can follow the loop back upward in a nature creation and form your own deities. Perhaps these deities are different than the prime moving Divine Source, but to the believer in natural creation they are just as real as the Singularity beyond.

The Whole

In Tantric philosophy, if anything is to exist, everything must exist. The male cannot exist without the female, nor could either exist without the spirit or the earth. Everything is important as a part of the Whole, and the Whole is the summation of everything.

It is often said that without black you would be unable to recognize white; but it is also true that without all the various colors in the multiverse, you would not be able to recognize color differences. Further, all color together might be thought of as black, whereas an absence of color might be thought of as white. Yet when we reverse the situation, we know that white light can be split into every color of the rainbow and that the total absence of light results (in our perception) in blackness.

For a total comprehension, we must understand this seeming paradox. In Tantra every emotion and every shade of emotion that you are capable of must be recognized. Every appetite you have must also be comprehended. There must be a time for stillness and an appreciation of stillness, and a time for motion and an appreciation of motion. Finally there must be understanding and comprehension of every step on the way from stillness to motion.

Once all the planet-plane comprehensions are gained, this comprehension is extended first to the spirit plane wherein the gods are metaphors of the comprehensions gained in the planet plane as applied to the spirit plane, and then past the spirit plane into the comprehension that the Beyond either contains all of the colors as in our white light, or none of the colors as in the white absence-of-color discussed above.

OFFERINGS

Tantra philosophy has come to incorporate the idea that you should propitiate the God-ess by making offerings. Traditionally such offerings have been differentiated into five major categories:

1) Offering to the God-ess the choicest piece of an animal recently slaughtered.

2) Offering choice selections of recently gathered crops or slaughtered animals to the animal representing the God-ess in a given chakra.

3) Offering inanimate yet valuable things to the God-ess, especially gold, silver, and jewels.

4) Offering the result of study on the path of a God-ess: perhaps a philosophical work, a poem or a song, or some similar result of study dedicated to the God-ess.

5) Offering to strangers physical or spiritual nourishment.

The offering is the giving up of something of value when you seek the intervention of the God-ess in earth-plane matters. The offering must be quite deliberate and must be done with appropriate reverence and ritual. You can develop these offerings for yourself. They are typical God-ess bargains of the most simple sort: "I do something for you, and you do something for me." We have all experienced this type of offering in our own lives: "My God, if you get me out of this situation, I'll go to church every Sunday for a month of Sundays."

WORSHIP

Worship in Tantra is more the contemplation or attentiveness to the idea behind a God-ess than saying prayers. It is subdivided into various levels of contemplation, with contemplation of the contemplation being the highest level. Typical levels of contemplation are of the world, of life, of spirit, of God-ess, of contemplation itself. When these are contemplated with the idea behind the picture of a particular God-ess, you are worshipping that God-ess.

This technique is designed to get you into all the aspects of each God-ess. Look at figure 23 on page 156, our very first Godess Dakini. To worship this type of savage, you must comprehend:

1) The need for the savage beginnings of our world or the universe, the big bang, the volcanic eruptions, the directed chaos.

2) The relationship of her primal feelings to your present life. The primal feelings we all suppress must be allowed to surface so you can understand their effect on your behavior and the essential part of you they form.

3) The place in the spiritual world held by creation. The relationship between the earth-microcosm and the spiritmacrocosm needs to be comprehended.

4) The place of this God-ess in the pantheon of God-esses in the macrocosm. Who is she? What is she? What is her relationship to you?

5) Whether you are a participant in a two-way exchange with the God-ess, or you are able to detach your spiritual entity and let "Me" understand the God-ess' feelings while "I" communes with the spirit of the God-ess. In other words, can you contemplate the interaction while being one with the spirit of the Godess?

ENTERING THE SPIRAL OF THE CHAKRAS

A trip through the chakras first takes you up through the natural, and then down through the divine. It is a circle or a continuous loop around which you can proceed until you leave it and enter the Beyond, either in death or through your Tantric discipline.

It is usual for gurus to start you out as we did—from the base chakra—and to bring you up through all the chakras and then down again to return to the place from which you started. However, on any given day you may come into chakric ritual, contemplation, and meditation at any level of consciousness. For instance, if you are feeling very "up," you would consider yourself to be in tune with the heart chakra. You can in fact enter the spiral at that level and move upward; however, experience has clearly shown that it is better when coming into the chakras to enter at your emotional level, then very quickly go down through the chakras without illuminating them, and start your contemplation in the base. The time spent in the chakras below your emotional level can be minimal; then very rapidly, gaining speed, you give yourself a running start at the remaining chakras above your emotional level to burst forth through the crown into the Beyond.

Compare your present emotional level with a schoolyard swing in a resting state. You are serene and content and you are lifted above yourself by sitting above the ground in the swing. With a lot of mental effort, you can make the swing sweep backward and upward. This is like going down through the chakras. At the peak of its rearward motion, the swing is released and given a strong push. Now as you come up through the chakras you gather tremendous momentum and pass the place where you were previously sitting. Your emotions rise and you leave the swing, as it goes over the top in a complete circle, heart and mind reaching for the vastness of the blue sky beyond. Stay as long as you can in the Beyond and then come back down until you are again resting at the place you started.

You have traveled from the base beyond the crown and returned again to the base. You have experienced an age-old journey that is hinted at in many mystical systems. The upward activation part of the journey has within it the secret for raising psychic power. This is the serpent power, so widely discussed but

so little understood. It is the power of Mother Nature represented by Shakti in all her aspects.

RAISING THE SERPENT

Just as the mushroom appears instantly in the night, and just as
the lingam instantly erects from nothing in the presence of
Shakti, so the snake arises from its coils to strike. In the mundane world, the beauty or the caress of Shakti in her lover
aspect causes the lingam to erect. The serpent kundalini lives in
the psychic world and Shakti's psychic presence makes the
snake suddenly, instantly straighten out. Imagine beating a
coiled cobra with a stick. The snake lying there lethargic suddenly straightens out.

If you have ever been at a fire and watched the coiled canvas
hose suddenly grow stiff and rigid under the impact of high-
pressure water, and then have seen a fireman wrestle the head to
keep it under control, you have some comprehension of how the
serpent suddenly straightens and spits forth its hiss. You can
ride the snake's head through the chakras and burst with its
hissing breath through the crown into the Beyond. The psychic
head of the serpent does not pass the secret chakra. Instead your
psyche rides its hiss into the beyond just as life rides with ejaculated semen into the yoni.

The power of the serpent as it uncoils its spring can be
directed outward into the world (in which case the serpent head
is pointed out through the brow chakra) or allowed to carry you
straight on upward into a new non-conceptual awareness of
reality. Wherever the serpent takes you, that is the place you
should be. When you have indwelt, you must remember to
bring yourself back down to the base so you can re-enter the
world with stability. To come suddenly into the reality of our
imperfect world after the encounter with the Singularity gives
your psyche an abrupt jolt. Many find it difficult to do mun-

dane work for months afterward—simply because they find it pointless and obnoxious to their new value system.

YOUR CONTINUOUS LOOP OF DEVELOPMENT

When you have climbed the chakras, gone as far as you can Beyond, and returned once, you have completed one psychic loop. The journey has empowered you to overcome your emotions, leave them behind, gain new knowledge, and bring that wisdom back with you. During the Kundalini Circle exercise, you progressively moved further into the Beyond. After you have experienced the full cycle two or three times, then during the Kundalini Circle you change your approach. As you enter the meditation phase, you are in the base chakra. Very quickly you let your mind and emotions run up through the chakras into the secret chakra and beyond, and then without waiting you run down again. Then you quickly repeat the cycle. The first cycle may take you 20 or 30 seconds. After several repetitions you will find you have speeded up until you can get through a cycle in less than ten seconds.

An easy way of thinking about the cycle is the progression of mantras shown in figure 39. Notice that the silent M is not sounded after the first mantras but only after the OM. If you

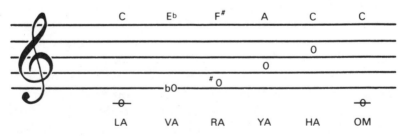

Figure 39.   How the mantras progress.

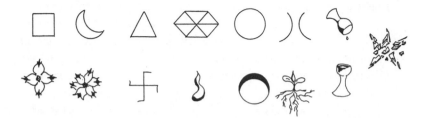

Figure 40. How the symbols progress.

think of yourself doing these notes more and more rapidly, eventually they might turn into almost a buzz. When you feel you are ready, hold onto the O<u>M</u> when you get it and move from the low O<u>M</u> to the high O<u>M</u> to the silent O<u>M</u>, while you think of riding the snake's head and then its hiss into the Beyond.

It may be that you are not into sounds and chants. If that is true, you might want to consider the succession of symbols shown in figure 40. First imagine they are individual slides being projected on the screen of your mind. Then they speed up and flicker like an old-fashioned movie projection. Now they blur

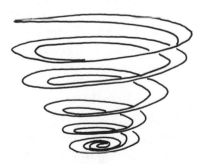

Figure 41.   Continuous loop of signposts.

and move together and become a continuous, moving, tangible thing that is the loops of the snake as it uncoils within you.

If you are not into either sound or symbols, you should go into the chakra signposts and decide which signpost turns you on the most. Then make your own continuous loop of signposts that will help you travel progressively faster and higher around the loop. The loop is shown in figure 41. Notice that it is actually a kind of mashed spiral. It starts as a circle and gradually its vertical dimension becomes more pronounced until suddenly it breaks as you leave this plane of understanding and move into the Beyond.

METHODS OF RAISING THE SERPENT

The ancient literature describes many other ways that are helpful in raising the serpent. If you have difficulty after sustained genuine effort, you may try some of them. These are not quick fixes but serious methods that will take you a lot of time to set up, experiment with, and use.

Beating

When you are sitting in meditation after completing two or three kundalini circles, lay a small wooden cylinder under the base of your spine. The cylinder should be about one foot long and perhaps three inches in diameter. Gently raise yourself and support your weight on the knuckles of both hands. Rhythmically beat your perineum on the cylinder while you mentally go through your cycle of chakras. The beating will awaken even a recalcitrant serpent.

Breathing

When you are sitting in meditation, close the head orifices with the fingers. Put your forefinger (index finger) on your eye, your thumb on your ear, and the ring finger on the side of your nose. Maintain a gentle but firm pressure. Start ha-tha breathing.

Slow down those deep breaths as much as you can while you continue to go through your chakra cycle. Eventually you will find a comfortable, very slow breathing level that you can maintain without conscious effort. At this point the serpent—who believes that its residence will be destroyed by death—rouses itself to bring you out of the trance.

Clenching

Two systems are used here:

For the single worker: Each time you come into the base chakra in your psychic loop, you first strain downward as if you are having a very difficult bowel movement; then you suck the anus back in. Someone watching your anus can help you in this exercise, because the anus does actually move inward and outward when the exercise is done correctly. The further you can make it move in and out, the more correct is the exercise. As you continue with your psychic loops, every time you come down into the base you push out and every time you move up from the base you suck in. This action near its lair rouses the serpent.

For the dyadic couple: In the female the forefinger is inserted into the yoni and the thumb into the posterior yoni. The two are rhythmically pressed together. This actually is pressing on the lair of the serpent. In the male, the thumb is inserted into the posterior yoni and the forefinger is pushed into the testicular sac (scrotum) and hooked into the bottom of the pelvic bone; then similar rhythmic squeezing is used.

Soma

Drinking a small amount of alcohol is often beneficial, provided the mind can still totally control the body without conscious effort. However, in some people even the smallest amount of alcohol interrupts the completion of the kundalini circle.

Other Methods

In their desperation, some people try for years to raise the serpent power. They try drugs, masochistic behavior, and bodily abuse of all kinds. All these activities are totally unnecessary. Do not try to make kundalini raise its head before you are ready for it. Following strict Tantric discipline you may be ready in four to six months, or it may take you longer. If you follow the discipline you will know, because each successive month you will recognize that you have reached new and different planes of understanding. As long as you are progressing, don't change anything. Be content. One of the big problems with modern life is the expectation of instant gratification and the timing of everything in milli- and micro-seconds. When the serpent is raised, it straightens and carries you in a flash of time; but the time needed to raise the serpent properly cannot be gauged on a linear time clock. Impatience is one of the bodily emotions that you MUST overcome before you can truly be one with the Singularity.

TRANSCENDING THE APPETITES

Tantra insists that natural impulses and desires are to be indulged in, studied, and overcome. Tantrists laugh at the ascetic because he or she has no comprehension of the pleasures of the world. There is no need for control if someone has no comprehension of a pleasure-experience. These ideas come directly from the very oldest writings on which Hinduism is based. Verse after verse in the Bhagavad Gita speaks of controlling the senses and the intelligence. Typically, in Book 3, Verse 33: "Beings follow their nature. What can repression accomplish?"

Overcoming and controlling the most exquisite pleasure lead to control of the mind. In the Maithunic practice, where the lingam is allowed to move within the yoni for a long time but orgasm does not occur, practitioners learn to control one of their most basic impulses—that of reproduction. In the later cycles of the Kundalini Circle, a new type of Maithuna is undertaken, in which the body pulses of a pseudo-orgasm occur but the semen is retained. This total control of the body by the mind is the object of the practice. Simultaneously with the control of orgasm, control of lowered breath and seen or felt perceptions are entered into. Nothing going on outside the body is allowed to influence the equanimity of the mind, as it contemplates one of the great truths or paradoxes of a given chakra. Conscious control of the process is the first step on the path.

After conscious control has been practiced for some time, the control becomes automatic and unconscious. In the first states of Maithunic practice, a conscious effort is required not to have an orgasm and to withdraw the lingam from the yoni knowing that it will be a long time before they are reintroduced to each other. After two or three experiences, it becomes easier, although still under conscious control. After six or eight experiences, there is nothing to it. It is the extension of such practice that allows the Indian fakir to lie on a bed of nails or to injure himself without feeling pain. Such practice, however, is specifically identified as negative in the Hindu scriptures. It is recognized as vanity and conceit and fanatic ostentation.

It is also pointed out that people who go on an austere diet often make their body weak, and that self-torture and bodily weakness together produce hallucinations which are often mistaken for spiritual visions. Control should not be confused with pain and torture. Total unconscious control of the senses and the autonomic nervous system is what is desired. All humans are victims of their own senses and impulses. It is these senses and impulses you must learn to control automatically. First you control them with the will and then you control them without thinking about it, remembering always that the senses must never be allowed to atrophy.

Westerners assume that they are the prisoners of their appetites; instead we should enjoy our appetites and make them our

servants. A typical familiar example is the use of anger in an
argument. To the Westerner, someone showing great anger must
have some form of right on his side, because "mature people
never lose control and get violently angry unless they are in the
right and have been wronged." There is a tendency, of course, to
move away from an angry person. The passionate emanations of
anger make most people feel uneasy. Thus if you USE anger you
can win an argument—but if you let anger be your master, your
mind will be incapable of logical thought; whereas if you make
anger your servant, it can be useful.

When you learned in earlier chapters to raise and send out
your power, you simulated emotions. In the same way you can
get into the mode of anger to the extent that you'll put out
power of such negativity that people will avoid you. In a difficult
situation, these emanations can be used as a protective force.
Instead of the fear you may be feeling, simulate anger. You will
be surprised how people avoid bugging you.

UNDERSTANDING AND RELINQUISHING

Once you grow comfortable with your friends in a Tantric
group, you will be able to let down the guard you put up
between yourself and the world. This will be almost a physical
releasing each time you rejoin the group from outside. As you
come in through the door it is as if you expelled a breath of pent-
up apprehension. You can now be yourself, free to say and do
anything and everything you want to. This relaxation is one of
the first stages in your search for awareness.

The next stage is reached when you recognize that the material possessions which you have collected and clung to through
your life are no longer important, either to yourself or to the
group of people whom you are with. You have relinquished your
materialistic drive. This is not to say you should not go out into
the world and get fair return for the work you do; it is just that
you have grown beyond the need to "own" things.

The writers of this book live under a vow of poverty, though they still appear to own many things: their clothing, their books, their trinkets. Perhaps they have a kind of lease on their use for a time, but the right to that lease is tentative at best. Call it custodial. When they die, their belongings will revert to a religious association. The motives that lead entrepreneurs, for instance, to pile up millions of tokens called dollars are quite incomprehensible to the authors. Native Americans could not comprehend the frontier assumption of land ownership or property ownership: "The land came down to us. It will go on to our children. It should not be divided or owned by anyone."

Another thing you will relinquish in your search for the Beyond is the thought that you will ever REACH the Beyond! For if you sit in breathless anticipation of some flash of awareness, or if you grind your teeth and say, "I am entitled to reach the Beyond!" the flash will never arrive. After you have waited eternally and become bored with it and are past the point where you would normally abandon something that seems to have failed, that is the moment when suddenly you will break through. In fact you may have given up the hope that it will work, but are continuing the effort for the sake of those around you.

The work and exercises you do must be a pleasure. When it becomes an onerous duty it certainly will not work. If you are watching a clock, waiting for this phase to be over, tapping your toe, you are going to get nowhere. If it becomes a duty, withdraw from the exercise until you can approach it as a pleasurable natural experience in itself and part of your whole life. In other words, live and enjoy a life as perfect in its cyclical rhythms as it could possibly be. When you have relinquished the expectation of reward and are enjoying the journey for itself, the destination will be there when it is ready for you. Suddenly you will come upon the goal.

APPENDICES

The Tantric Kin
and House

The surviving scriptures of all ancient philosophies contain descriptions of realms in the spiritual world. By the microcosm/macrocosm commonality principle, "As above, so below," the spiritual world is identical in structure to the world in which we live. In our ongoing research into the spiritual world,[1] we have found that spiritual realms are still recognizable from ancient philosophical descriptions, easily equated to several ancient philosophies, and readily correlated with the chakras. Table 6 on page 269 shows this commonality of realms. Read it carefully; for though the similarities are quite striking, the entries are not exact equivalents.

In our work and in ancient philosophy, we found that just as Ida and Pingala meet and intertwine, so spirits of diverse backgrounds have to meet, reconcile, and meld in the spiritual before the combined spirit can progress to higher realms.

You learned earlier that reincarnation is a progressive upward system. We are here on this plane of existence to grow and to learn all we can about ourselves and the world in which we live. It is clear that this process continues after death. In order to avoid many repetitive incarnations, you should work on this plane to learn those things that will allow you to pro-

---

[1]Gavin and Yvonne Frost, *Astral Travel* (York Beach, ME: Samuel Weiser, 1986).

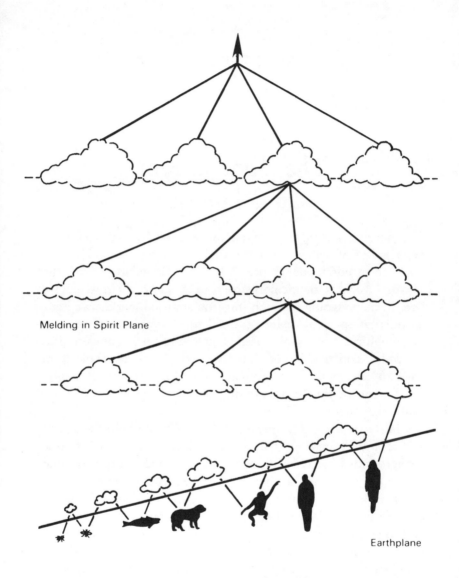

Melding in Spirit Plane

Earthplane

Figure 42.   Progression on the Earth plane and in realms above. In each Earth incarnation, we progress both spiritually and evolutionarily. So the smallest bug can eventually evolve into human consciousness—and each time the "spirit matter" grows. You eventually leave the Earth plane to meld with other spirits.

Table 6. Comparison of Spiritual Realms

Egyptian	Qabalah	Tarot	Modern Name	Chakra
The One	Crown	Fool	The place we cannot think of	Crown
Judgment	Understanding	World	Last Gate	Brow
Maat	Wisdom/ Justice	Judgment	Judgment	Throat
Fire	Love	Sun	Variable	Heart
Sekhet Aaru	Beauty	Tower	Cultural	Navel
Hapi	Glory	Temperance	Here-Now	Pelvic
Tua'i	Victory	Death	The World	Base

gress most rapidly through the various stages in both present and future levels of reincarnation. After "death," when a spirit no longer needs to return to this plane of existence, it melds with other similar spirits who have achieved high development before it progresses onward toward IT from which all spirits originate.

From various experiments we have done with astral-traveling subjects, it appears that several advanced spirits meld into one. Figure 42 on page 268 shows this process of reincarnation, both on the earth plane and in the spiritual world. When it first passes permanently into the spiritual world, the spirit still has much to learn. It's ready to move up — yet still contains many earth-plane ideas such as ego and petty emotions. It gets rid of these by melding with other spirits or by a learning process which is a continuation of that which it has already undergone. First male and female spirits merge, losing gender identity. Then people of different cultures merge, losing cultural identity. This seems to show that gender differences are easier to lay aside than cultural ones.

Tantrists believe that each spirit melds with three other spirits before progressing to the next plane of existence; and that this melding process is repeated at least four times before the spirit can rejoin IT. Just as the joining of the male and the female on the earth plane creates the yin-yang completeness, so the melding of one person with three others is an earth-plane equivalent of the melding that is to come on the other side of the Invisible Barrier.

Tantrists believe that the melding is designed to subordinate the individual self to the Whole. A key function of a Tantric house is to teach its members selflessness and willing melding with others, especially those of different racial and cultural backgrounds.

In the melding process each spirit surrenders part of its individuality to the new Whole, the larger spirit. Thus in order to meld quickly, the spirit must have a high degree of selflessness. Selflessness can be learned on this plane of existence, and it is most easily learned by giving up personal possessions, including the "possession" of a lover or spouse. Tantrists can develop this selflessness in their living arrangements, first in a Tantra house and then in the larger ashram.

EMOTIONS AND LOVE

In the Western world, the agape love idea promulgated by the entertainment industry and by romance novels has led many to believe that sexual intercourse is an inseparable part of loving another person. To the Tantrist this is a laughable concept. Sexual intercourse is for pleasure, for adjusting hormone levels, for removing tensions, for producing children, and for creating the macrocosm in the microcosm. Love is a relationship that may or may not have a sexual connotation. The mother and the father love a child; brothers and sisters love one another; married sexually active partners often hate each other and have nothing but the bed in common. In many Western minds "fuck" is a dirty word; moreover, it often carries the connotation of hostility between the partners. Thus a phrase like, "I love her and I'm gonna fuck her brains out," is meaningless and contradictory. Tantrists do not confuse loving with lusting, or with sexual intercourse, or with learning selflessness.

Various Tantric rituals require sexual intercourse and contact. If you cannot or will not have sex with another member of the house, you must honestly examine with that other member the reasons for the problem. If he or she has a habit that to you is gross and repulsive, you should honestly tell of your revulsion. On the other hand, it may be faulty training or something within your own mind that says, "I cannot do sex without love." All the members of a house should love each other. They all should work to help each other develop. More love exists between the members in a house than exists between many married couples; but it is not the wide-eyed calf-love of song and story. A Tantric definition of love might be "the wish to see another develop to his or her fullest potential."

What if you are deeply "in love" with another person and you both join a Tantra house? You must give up your possessive attitude toward the other person. What if, in order to develop, one of you needs to take a job or attend a university in a distant place? The parting may be painful, but through the pain you learn selflessness and develop.

You learned earlier how raising the force is enhanced by the controlled use of sexual differences, and how emotional control is gained through the control of sex. In a Tantric group, sex is used for many purposes, such as overcoming your ego and possessiveness (both of other people and of personal property), and learning through multiple coupling with others how the macrocosm can be brought to the microcosm.

THE HOUSE AND THE ASHRAM

In figure 42 (on page 268) you saw that in the melding process different numbers of spirits are melded together to form larger entities. Table 7 shows these numbers at each level of progression. This explains why Tantrists strive toward having sixteen members in a house. If any group is to represent perfectly the macrocosm in the microcosm, it must contain the correct number of people. Thus a minimum house contains four and an ideal "perfect" house contains sixteen working adults; a minimum ashram 64, and an ideal ashram 256. When a house or an ashram passes perfection, it splits. It is our belief that the reason several large ashrams failed was the fact that they did not observe this simple rule. The Rajneesh ashram in Oregon had exceeded the limit of manageability a hundredfold and had to fail.

In some houses the memory of the numbers is reinforced by doing all the work of the kundalini cycle together in the exercise room. As with all things, the guru recommends you try it and see whether it feels natural and good to your house. The use of a roster for partner changes and a fairly rigid system of work and play seem to focus attention on the purpose of the ritual and away from "free sex."

JOINING THE TANTRIC HOUSE

When you first transform your own house into a Tantric house by having another couple join you, all that will happen logisti-

Table 7. The Macrocosm in the Microcosm

Melding Level	Spirits Melded	Tantric Earth Plane
1	4	Minimum House
2	16	Ideal House
3	64	Minimum Ashram
4	256	Ideal Ashram

cally is that you will adjust the living space to the requirements of Tantra. Soon, however, you will want others to join so you can extend your development. We make two suggestions:

1) Do not invite people in too quickly.

2) Invite only people who have a thorough knowledge of the meaning and practice of Tantra.

If you are not careful, all you will get is people hoping for cheap thrills and lots of (wow) sex. They will give your house a bad reputation and will take more than they give. When you do finally find a single person or a couple who wishes to join the house—who have taken theoretical training for at least six months—the new member should be brought in only on probation and should do the following:

1) Sign an undertaking with the house that he or she will pay the fair share of support for the period of probation;

2) Have a complete physical to make sure he or she has no communicable diseases;

3) Fill out a family medical history questionnaire to learn whether any new member has diseases that can be transmitted genetically.

All people invited to join must be well-adjusted non-parasitic members of society. Tantra is not for people who are looking for an escape from the world or who cannot make it in the world. There are many easier ways to get sex; and there are social service agencies intended to provide welfare. Free-loaders and sexual athletes bring nothing but grief to your group.

If present members of the house cannot comfortably fulfill ritual requirements with the new probationers, adjustments must be made. After an honest discussion of the probationer's problems and an honest attempt by the probationer to overcome any problems, if the probationer still cannot be assimilated comfortably, the probationer should be rejected.

The members of the house who cannot accept the probationer owe it to themselves to get their feelings into the open—
for it may be shortcomings in their own development that cause
this rejection of the probationer, rather than a flaw in the probationer. The self-analysis should happen as early as possible in
the probationary period, remembering always that one "no"
vote at the end of the probationary period means the probationer is rejected and must leave the house. During the probation period, depending on house rules, the candidates may or
may not take part in the standard roster of ritual and work.
These should be fixed rules, not changed when some "hunk" or
"doll" enters the house.

The probationary period lasts from six months to a year.
After the probation, successful candidates become fully initiated
priests and priestesses of Tantra. At this point they take a vow of
poverty, committing all their mundane earnings and all their
worldly possessions to the house.

Admission to full house membership is voted on by all
present adult members. At this stage any present member is
entitled to blackball probationers. No reasons need be given and
the identity of the blackballing member is not revealed. Members should not be argued into accepting a new member they
don't like or whom they feel uneasy about, for harmony in the
house is of the highest importance.

Remember: There is often a problem before probationers
adjust to the rhythms of the house, and house members learn
quickly to adjust to the high sex drive of probationers during
their first two or three months in an open society. In the first
days of probation, high drives are natural.

Before letting a new member join your house, clearly tell
him or her that no member of a Tantra house ever has sexual
relations with anyone outside the house. This is one of the very
few absolute taboos in Tantra, and is based, of course, on the
existence of sexually transmitted diseases in the outside world.
Moreover, those entering a house are making a commitment to
it. If you find someone you love in the outside world, you may

teach that person Tantra and maybe after one or two years, the partner will be admitted to the house. Thus the commitment to the house sometimes presents a temporary problem to one of its members.

THE MARE AND THE HARE

Occasionally a new probationer must be rejected because his or her genitalia are either much larger or much smaller than the average in the house. The term "well hung" is the Western equivalent of what the Kama Sutra calls a horse man; and unless all the male members of the house are well endowed, a single horse probationer should ideally not be admitted. Nor should the male who is drastically under-endowed (the hare) be admitted—to THIS house. The biggest problem of all, however, is not to gauge this by the males of the house but to gauge it by the females. It is not generally realized in the West that some yonis are very large and others are small. The large, or elephant, yoni may be incapable of tightening to the extent that the quintessential pleasure can be achieved from it by any but a horse man, and a deer, or small yoni, woman experiences more pain than pleasure from the various rituals if her partner is too large. As in the case of the males,

Table 8. Equal and Unequal Unions

Equal		Unequal	
Man	Woman	Man	Woman
Hare	Deer	Hare	Mare
Bull	Mare	Hare	Elephant
Horse	Elephant	Bull	Deer
		Bull	Elephant
		Horse	Deer
		Horse	Mare

females with major yonic variations should be rejected before they are accepted as probationers. The Kama Sutra defines these variations in the following way:

Man is divided into three classes, viz., the hare man, the bull man, and the horse man.

Woman also, according to the depth [and width] of her yoni, is either a deer, a mare, or an elephant.

There are thus three equal unions between persons of corresponding dimensions, and six unequal unions when the dimensions do not correspond, or nine in all. These are shown in Table 8 on page 275.

THE YOUNG, THE OLD, AND THE UGLY

It is found in the Western house that age differences can cause problems during ritual. Even though the older member may be fully capable and have a well-exercised lingam or yoni, younger members may be repulsed simply because of the age difference (and the assumed unattractiveness of an "older" person). This problem has to be overcome in the minds of younger members. Once sexual maturity is reached, there should be no problem doing ritual with partners of any age, although Tantrists do try to keep their house within an age range as narrow as possible simply because the interests of the various people at different age levels is different. Older people may want to listen to opera when the youngsters would rather dance to rock music. These differences in taste have little or nothing to do with the time spent in ritual exercises, where all are intent on a common goal. Most real people are short on glamor, and few are Playboy/girl centerfolds; but this makes little difference to their dedication or performance in ritual. In fact, people aware of their shortcomings often make up for them by being better at ritual performance than those who think themselves beautiful and desirable, who in the outside world are accustomed to trading on good looks.

A WORD ABOUT CHILDREN

Infants and young children adjust readily to nudist living and the loving behavior among the adult residents of a Tantric house. They think nothing of the fact that they see adults doing exercises and rituals together which include the placing of the lingam into the yoni. They happily crawl and walk around "heaven-clad" and enjoy skin-to-skin contact with others in affectionate hugs. Children who have attended a conventional kindergarten or the early grades in public school sometimes have more difficulty in adjusting to the house; and candidates who have children of 7 or older are often not accepted into a house. Once children reach their maturity at age 18, they may study Tantra and join a house; and of course they are welcome in the house of their mother, where they have the option of participating in rituals. Thus there exists a near-taboo on taking into a house children between the ages of 7 and 18 and their parents, though of course each case must be evaluated on its own merits. There is no hard and fast taboo; but as a student of Tantra, you should be aware of the potential problem.

KEEPING PETS

No animals are kept by Tantrists because they believe the caging of an animal, even in an area as large as a house, is wrong and more importantly that all their loving and caring instincts should be focused on the other people in the house.

THE DYADIC COUPLE

Within a balanced Tantra house (where numbers of yogis and of yogins are equal), a simple straightforward roster is established so that every two months at full moon the assigned ritual couples change partners. This is a regularly scheduled change containing no surprises to anyone and no favoritism. In a house which is temporarily unbalanced, the roster is more difficult to arrange, and it is usual for roster changes to occur more frequently. In these instances, two of one gender are partnered with one of the other for a maximum of one month.

The usual arrangement is the couple. These are called "dyadic" pairs because they are dedicated to remaining a couple for the duration of the specified roster and performing all ritual acts together for that time. This is not to say they are forbidden from making love with others; only that they must be available and to the best of their ability fulfill their ritual obligations with their assigned partner for the period of time specified by the roster.

During their assigned time together they are responsible not only for ritual matters but also for the care, grooming, and general well-being of their partner. In the purification rituals they scrub the skin of the partner. They also do such things as combing each other's hair, aiding in the removal of skin blemishes, being honest with the partner to help overcome bad habits, and supporting the partner in time of need. This grooming and caring for each other includes not only the mundane body, but also the psychic body; so psychic healing procedures are often used by one partner on the other.

Nor is the mundane neglected. Full dyadic partnership includes shopping together or handling mundane needs. Sometimes dyadic partners who have vastly different views and backgrounds spend hours discussing their differences and pooling knowledge of skills. All of this is growth. Growth ceases when the partnership becomes one-sided; when one partner gives and supports, and the other takes and becomes dependent. Each must give thought to the other. Each must give physical support and help to the other. A house cannot long exist when even one of its members is selfish. The dyadic relationship is meant to teach equality, fairness, selflessness. All this requires the subordinating of selfish wishes. Sometimes, for example, a yogin brings her partner to orgasm even though she does not want to complete the experience herself. This is a perfectly acceptable thing in a Tantric house—provided that when she feels like it, her partner should bring her to climax without climaxing himself, so she knows he is doing it for her wishes, not just out of selfish lust.

There is a widespread folk belief that when a man gets an erection it is somehow dangerous or harmful to let that erection deflate without ejaculating. This is a simple folk belief, and perhaps is reinforced by exploitive males who have in mind the benefits to be gained by themselves. It is true that when an untrained student maintains his erection for several hours, muscular pain can result; but this is simply a tired-muscle pain that does no physical damage. It is true that after a certain point is reached (very late in sexual play), it is better for an ejaculation to occur than not. This is also true of the female. If she is brought to a certain point of arousal where the whole experience becomes very one-pointed, the act should be completed; hence the Tantric taboo on interrupting any couple in their more private moments.

WHAT A TANTRIST WEARS

When going into the outside world, Tantrists dress so they will not be noticed. They do not waft around in Indian saris, multiple layers of see-through veils, or garlands of blossoms. They dress inconspicuously because they are not using their attire to make a statement outside the house. Their statement is made by the way they treat others and by the achieving life they live in the business community. As we have said, Tantrist couples tend to shop for clothes in the dyadic mode. Occasionally one member of a Tantric house will have a very capable eye for attire. This person should always be consulted in choices of attire.[2]

---

[2]Some very simple rules are occasionally violated. If you enjoy dressing in vivid colors, do not add garish jewelry to such attire. If you like to wear conspicuous jewelry, wear garments in quiet colors.

Learn from the mistakes of others, and aim for quiet good taste while remaining true to yourself.

Within the house dress varies depending on the region of the house you are in. Conventional work clothes are worn in the public parlor area. In the leisure area they are laid aside in favor of a light cotton knee-length tunic-like caftan. For most of the month total nudity is observed in all bedrooms, bathrooms, and ritual exercise areas.

During the month, sexual activity varies from none in the time near the new moon to a maximum at full moon. In the time of new moon (which is also the time of the females' menstruation) all members wear a dhoti. This simple garment is made from a single piece of fabric that goes around the waist, down at the back, up in the front, and hangs apron-like over the genitalia. The dhoti serves several purposes: the difference between menstruating and non-menstruating females is minimized; during this time of no intercourse, control or lack of control of the lingam in exercise periods is hidden, saving distraction on everyone's part. If the house is such that no females menstruate, the requirement for the dhoti can be dropped.

In summary, there are no hard and fast dress codes in Tantra. Sensible, conservative, non-provocative attire is the aim. When cooking and eating, sex play is inappropriate. When outside the house, attracting attention through attire is also inappropriate.

ARRANGING THE CYCLES OF REGULATED, CONTROLLED SHARING

The Tantrist relies on ritual as a firm basis of life. The schedule is regulated by the long-term cycles of the moon and the sun. Although the smooth flow of these long-term cycles is occasionally interrupted by people joining and leaving the house, or by problems that arise, still the ritual continues. As the members of the house grow older and fewer surprises occur, even changes caused by human nature are smoothed out. Sudden changes of assignment are disruptive, so work and ritual rosters should be scheduled months or even years in advance. Assignments of ritual partners should last two months per dyad; for older well-established houses, three months is considered better.

Underlying the ritual assignments are the tasks required for running the house. No matter how much one person loves cooking or gardening, he or she should never be assigned a favorite chore forever. The tasks should be rotated to let everyone take a turn. It is usual for task assignments to be changed over at the minimum-work time, or full moon, and tasks are assigned to dyads on a monthly basis so dyads get a change of pace. All tasks are assigned so that balance is maintained; in other words, even in heavy chores equal numbers of males and females do the work.

The normal separation of tasks falls into the following general categories: cooking, dishwashing/purchasing, laundry and housework, yardwork. These chores can be traded off among members, for instance when a member is on shift work outside the house; however, eventually a balance must be achieved so that everyone gets a chance to clean the bathroom and everyone cooks (no matter how poorly) for the whole house. Dishwashing usually combines with purchasing provision for the house.

DESIGNING THE HOUSE

Many Tantrist houses start with two couples who want to get together and start a house. These two couples normally can live in a standard American dwelling, especially one of the large older residences in various city areas that are presently run down but are being rediscovered. These large older buildings can often be bought inexpensively and refurbished into extremely valuable and attractive homes that are very comfortable for two or more families to live in. Eventually, though, the

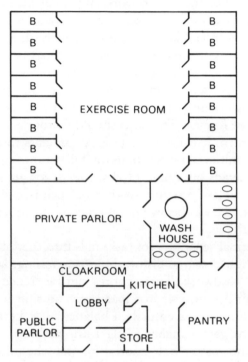

Figure 43. Simplified house layout. B = bedroom.

group will outgrow such living arrangements and will want their own specially designed house; then when the house becomes full in its turn they want to expand into the full ashram or community. The ultimate aim is always the ashram. It is the light at the end of the tunnel that beckons the Tantrist along.

You will derive much pleasure from designing your own house and making it comfortable. The plan shown in figure 43 naturally divides itself into two; many Tantric houses have two stories with areas for bathing, ritual, and exercise upstairs and general living quarters downstairs. The figure shows the layout of a house 50 x 80 feet intended for sixteen adults. This plan has no spaces for children, because children should have their own sleeping dormitory and play areas.

Some features of the house are interesting. For example, the walls of most rooms are built to a ratio of what is called the Golden Section or 0. When converted to feet and inches, the Golden Section ratios commonly used are as shown in Table 9 on page 284. For centuries it has been known that when buildings are designed with the walls in this ratio of 1.612 to 1, people are more comfortable living in them and they simply feel better.

The large exercise room can be a roofed-over, glass-walled, shed-like structure nestled in the L of an otherwise solid-walled house. If possible, the ritual exercise area should extend to an outdoor garden area which is not overlooked by neighbors. If it is not possible to arrange an outdoor area, appropriate sunlamps should be set up in the exercise area. There should be trees planted in the corners of this room, and the floor should be of wood covered with soft matting such as Japanese tatami mats. Around the wall spaces there should be eight low benches covered in a soft cotton fabric easily removable for laundering. Benches are usually of dimensions convenient for sexual activity (18 inches from the floor, 32 inches front to back, and 6 feet 6 inches long). A second set of these benches in bare wood of smaller dimensions is in the bath house.

At first glance, the sleeping rooms seem small by Western standards. Each contains a ³/₄ width long mattress, a lockable closet, a wash basin, a comfortable relaxing chair, a desk, and a desk chair. The desk is well lighted for study purposes. At the head of each bed is a buzzer connected to the door button and to a universal alarm system. Anyone seeking entry to the room must announce his or her presence, and the occupant may open the door or not; absolute privacy is thus assured. At no time is anyone entitled to question whether or not you were even in the room when they wanted access to you. Some emergency code signal is connected to the alarm buzzer system so that room occupants can all be warned simultaneously of any emergency that may occur.

Table 9. Ratios That Yield Ø

One Side	Other Side
8	5
16	10
32	20
48	30
64	40
80	50

This room is your own private space. You may be alone in it as long as you choose. Of course you must meet your ritual and work agenda; but otherwise you may do as you like. You may decorate it in any way you choose; though if it is too garish or heavily scented, you may be sure some other member will feel free to comment on your taste.

The bathroom or bath house is one of the most carefully designed rooms in the entire house. The central hot tub is its focus. A tub of 7 feet diameter and 4 feet deep is pleasant for sixteen people. Arranged outside the hot tub are washing benches. The procedure is for each person to dip up a bucket of water from the hot tub and use it to wash thoroughly as described in the purification rituals of chapter 5, aided by their dyadic partner. After thorough soaping and washing, they tip a bucket of water over themselves to remove most of the suds. Then they enter the hot tub. There is a prescribed squatting ritual that each does as he or she enters the tub, to make sure that the genitalia and anus are properly rinsed. After the squatting, members sit in the hot tub and soak up its beneficial heat.

Close to the bathroom, but separated from it by a wall of half-height, is a row of toilets. These are separated from each other again by walls of half height. The whole toilet area is tiled for good sanitary cleaning. It is separated from the bath area because the water play that often occurs around the hot tub may be disruptive in the toilet area. Hand-wash basins and mirrors are provided on the side nearest the dining area for those who must make up or do minor cosmetic adjustments before they go to work. Closets are provided just inside the dining area for storage of work clothing. The whole of the bath house floor, its walls, and the steps approaching the hot tub are finished in bare scrubbed wood, so no oils should be brought into the area.

The dining area and the kitchen are conventional. A single long table is used for dining; its upper surface is scrubbed bare wood. There is a bar between the kitchen and the dining room, and the kitchen wall is brought down from the ceiling so the exhaust fan can pull kitchen odors and smoke out of the house before they get into the dining room. Two four-burner stoves with ovens usually provide adequate cooking surfaces for eight couples. A deep-freeze and two large refrigerators are used together with a restaurant-style dishwasher.

Microwave ovens are not included because the effect of their emanations on psychic development seems to be negative. Further, if house members include women in their reproductive years or small children, the least bit of microwave radiation can damage their ova.

Two living rooms are included in the design. One, the public parlor, is for relaxed TV and music type living. It is large enough so that two TV sets can be housed. The other one is more a library than a living room. It is for contemplation, reading, and study. Many Tantra houses discourage any discussion of problems or decision-making during meals. Light conversation is perfectly acceptable; though many find that silence (especially at breakfast) helps them for the rest of the day. Books for reading and study are encouraged at all times; the more widely-read and knowledgeable the members, the better.

The garden deserves a special word. It is usually fenced in, and in warm climates must have plenty of shaded areas. It tends toward the Japanese rather formal low-maintenance design. A fountain and a flowing stream add to the serenity. The garden typifies the Yoga rule, "Out of chaos gradually is formed Order and through Order is formed the Spirit." The garden will take on a form and spirit reflecting the form and the spirit of the house; any newcomer should be warned that moving even one stone is forbidden until he has been in the house for at least a year.

Although some garden tools will be useful, after the original arrangement is complete, only simple hand tools should be retained. Along one side of the house there are protection and covered storage for the various house vehicles, and a very small and simple workshop. Everything in the house is made in as simple a way as possible. There is very little clutter, and no personal belongings are on display in the various shared rooms. It is best to start with absolutely bare, stark rooms and only gradually decorate the shared rooms by agreement of all members. There are no shelves, cupboards, or fussy little curtains to gather dust and make the house look cluttered. All ornaments are kept in natural shades, and as many as possible should be objects from nature. Garish paintings insult the eye of the Tantrist. Any new ornament should be placed in the meditation area of the library living room for at least three months before it is taken into the body of the house.

The parlor is used for meetings with visitors from the outside world: relatives, friends, and business people. Only very understanding relatives are allowed as far as the dining area, and none are allowed past that point; thus a separate toilet facility is required at the cloak room near the front door.

Tantra Supplement For Gay Students

by Glenn Malec

Tantra was devised as a heterosexual system, but does that mean it could not be adapted to homosexual use? No! Gay men and women occupy unique positions in the human species. Gay persons embody both male and female to such an extent that they do not seek members of the opposite gender for sexual unions. While a bi-sexual person does require the opposite gender, even if only on occasion, the truly gay person does not. It is not the purpose of this supplement to delve into the whys, but rather to show how Nirvana may be reached by the gay student of Tantra.

Refer to the following notes and instruction when studying the corresponding chapters for clarification to your lifestyle and the Tantrist path. Not all chapters require significant changes for use by gay students. If a specific chapter is not mentioned, it is because the student can put in any necessary changes without further help from me.

Mainstream gay relationships do not exist in a dominant/ subservient mode, but rather one of equality and sharing. To walk in balance, we must share in duties and tasks. This makes the partnership succeed. When you are able to help your lover/

partner, and it's mutual, you will continue to grow and strengthen together. Any other type of relationship will not work on the Tantrist path.

In these days of AIDS consciousness, an AIDS test would be a requirement for any person who wishes to join a Tantrist house. As all members are found AIDS-free and also free of any other contagious or sexually transmitted diseases, all the rituals can be performed without fear.

NOTES FOR CHAPTER 1

Being gay is natural and normal if this is the way you feel. This is very important to realize. Because conventional religions have put down women and gays for centuries, a lot of deprogramming and re-educating needs to be done. The general public is blasted about the "evils" of homosexuality and lesbianism. This stems from fear and from the desire to control others. The "sin" of sex has brainwashed many good people. Sex is natural, as is the enjoyment of it.

Tantrist Path

As everyone recognizes, the ability to do a sexual act with one's partner does not guarantee that it results in the maximum pleasure. Someone who is different and skilled can be a help in realizing maximum pleasure. This applies to all sexual preferences.

The Tantrist has no belief in the spiritual authority of a civil marriage. Some gays seek to legalize their relationship, but the orthodox Tantrist does not legalize a spiritual matter. The person whose spirit is advanced must have the freedom to advance further by associating with another of his or her own level.

The Tantrist path does not advocate promiscuity, but rather sexual contacts between consenting adults in private, and within a carefully selected and trained group. Gay relationships don't have the divorce problems to settle before forming their own house or entering a Tantrist house. There is no place for tears or sadness in Tantra. Even if you must sever a relationship to progress, do it, because you harm yourself by halting your own progress.

Sexual Notes

Because gay males have no true yoni to work with, the posterior yoni is used as a symbolic yoni. Remember that insertion is to be done by the partner who assumes the top role, as in the sunrise service. This symbolizes a mutual involvement. For the insertion use a water-based lubricant that cleans up quickly and completely.

Women have no true lingam to work with, so a double-sided artificial phallus can be used as the symbolic lingam. Each woman inserts her own side of the phallus in such as the sunrise service. Clean the phallus with plenty of soap and hot water after each use.

Only when both partners are actually joined in sexual union is there completion. Bliss can be achieved only when the need for maleness and the need for femaleness are removed. With gay Tantrists this is removed only when two compatible partners are joined.

Sexual needs must be fulfilled. The gay male, with the aid of his partner, must maintain the erect lingam to fulfill perfectly the ritual requirements. At the same time, he is not ridiculed if the erection cannot be maintained. Only he and his partner will know that this time they did not attain fullness. Partial coalescence is attained if the partners press the lingam against the posterior yoni while they maintain a deeply penetrating kiss with tongues touching.

Nirvana cannot be achieved when lust is present. All lust must be erased. This holds true no matter what your sexual preference is.

The Lingam

While a Playgirl or Mandate photo spread is enough to get many
a gay man an erection, you can lose this ease of erection in later
life or when you are over-exposed to such photos. The male
must remember how to do it and keep the erecting muscles
exercised. If, by following the instructions in chapter 1, you
cannot get an erection by will alone, your partner may help by
gently massaging the lingam. In lubricating the lingam, the oil
and lanolin massaging is done by the partner.

The Yoni

Glycerin and lanolin are the lubrication for the yoni. This internal application is gently done by the partner.

The male posterior yoni must also be given proper care.
Above all, the area must be kept clean and lightly lubricated.
Use water-based lubricants, because they are very easy to
remove.

Sunrise Ritual for Men

After cleaning in the morning as described on page 21, Male A
lies on the exercise mat with his hands toward the sun. Male B
lubricates Male A's lingam. Male B next takes the astride position with the lingam vitae completely encased in the posterior
yoni. Male A brings his knees up so that the flat soles of his feet
are together and places his hands above his head with palms
together. In this position the soles of Male B's feet are under
Male A's thighs. Male B places his hands outspread with palms
upward. He tips his head slightly backward and tightens his
pectoral muscles. Male A positions his hands so that the fingertips rest lightly on Male B's chest, then replaces his hands above
his head. They both take two full, deep breaths. Male B firmly
contracts his posterior yoni eight times in slow succession. In
response and in time with him, Male A enlarges the lingam.
With his right hand, Male B welcomes the sun by indicating in

turn each of the four chakras near the head, the throat, the heart, the genitalia. As he does this he says, "Father, I understand the health the sun will bring to me. Bless you for growing the food I will eat today. Let my heart send strength through my body to do your will. Beloved Mother of all, be happy the earth receives the sun."

When the affirmations are complete, Male B leans down and rests his forehead on Male A's forehead. To help this, Male A places his hands behind his neck and lifts his head. They both say, "Partner to partner, all is well. Good morning." (These are the first words they have spoken to anyone that day.) Male B dismounts and lies in the nesting position on the opposite side from which he usually sleeps with Male A, and they snuggle. A nesting of eight minutes is observed before sex play commences.

Sunrise Ritual for Women

Female A sits on the exercise mat, inserts one side of the phallus into her yoni, then lies back with her hands toward the sun. Female B takes the astride position encasing the artificial lingam in her yoni. Female A brings her knees up so that the flat soles of her feet are together and places her hands above her head with palms together. In this position the soles of her feet are under Female A's thighs. Female B places her hands outspread with palms upward. She tips her head slightly backward and lifts her breasts with her pectoral muscles. Female A positions her hands above her head. They both take two full, deep breaths. Female A and Female B both firmly contract each yoni eight times in slow succession and in unison. With her right hand, Female B welcomes the sun by indicating in turn each of the four chakras near the head, the throat, the heart, the genitalia. As she does this she says, "Father, I understand the health the sun will bring me. Bless you for growing the food I will eat today. Let my heart send strength through my body to do your will. Beloved Mother of all, be happy that the earth receives the sun."

When the affirmations are complete, Female B leans down and rests her forehead on Female A's forehead. To help this, Female A places her hands behind her neck and lifts her head. They both say, "Partner to partner, all is well. Good morning." (These are the first words they have spoken to anyone that day.) Female B dismounts and Female A removes the phallus. Female B then lies in the nesting position on the opposite side from which she usually sleeps with Female A, and they snuggle. A nesting of eight minutes is observed before sex play commences.

NOTES FOR CHAPTER 2

Maximizing the Force

For this experiment, try with various partners to see with whom you get maximum effect.

For the three-day experiments on page 31:

Day 1: Do the figure 4a experiment. Then hug and kiss your partner until both of you are sexually aroused. Repeat the experiment. Bring the lingam into contact with your partner's lingam, or your yoni into contact with your partner's yoni. Back off and repeat the experiment.

Men: Allow Male A's lingam to enter Male B's posterior yoni and make some motion.

Women: Place the artificial lingam (phallus) with each end into the respective yonis and make some motion.

When both partners are close to orgasm, back off and repeat the experiment. Follow with Day 2 and 3 in accordance with the chapter.

Which partner is A or B should be determined in advance for all services and experiments. Alternating A and B can be most rewarding since you can be in both roles.

NOTES FOR CHAPTER 4

Lotus-Stem Meditation

Men: Sitting with his back perfectly vertical and with his dyadic partner close by as on page 72, Male A directs his detailed concentration on Male B's lingam. First it is visualized as erect, ready, with the foreskin drawn back so that the head with its typical mushroom shape is seen. The same is visualized by Male B to Male A. Each partner thinks carefully of all details in turn, examining the hard, vibrant condition and the smooth baby-skin texture of the lingam. The texture is experienced as though it were touching the tongue or the tongue were exploring it. In the interior eye, the feeling of the tongue rubbing against the stem is experienced. Thus the stem is not felt with the finger but only with the tongue.

Now the male smell is brought to mind. In India, the incense patchouli is used on the lingam before sacred coupling. If you cannot bring the essence of the male to mind, imagine patchouli instead. The fact that this scent is indelibly imprinted on your consciousness in association with pleasurable sexual activity will intensify the effectiveness of the meditation.

Experience now the sound of the lingam. Its throbbing beat is faster than the deep earth tones of the Mother. It is insistent. It is sharp. It will not go away until it slowly melds with your own earth tones.

Now experience the vibrant thrusting nature of the lingam. If you like, imagine it inside you: its thrusting vibrancy, the male sword of pleasure, the essence of the male creative aspect. The feeling is one of the sun's heat and life.

One-pointed meditation can bring the experienced Tantrist right to the point of climax. At this point, a single touch to the underside of the lingam would push the yogi into climax. Practice this single-pointed meditation for longer and longer periods of time so that a single touch will bring the desired climax. The

intent of the meditation is to get to the point of climax and stay
there.

Women: Sitting with her back perfectly vertical, each dyadic
partner directs her detailed concentration to the yoni, visualizing it in all six of its aspects. It is pictured usually with the
brightest of labia, the clitoris vibrant and healthy, erect, and the
vagina itself gently opening and closing like a flower, inviting
entry. Clearly if the artificial phallus touches this opening and
closing yoni, it will be sucked in gently but firmly.

The texture of the yoni is next experienced, soft and warm,
moist and welcoming. Then each partner concentrates on the
scent of the feminine essence. During the sacred rites, a little
musk is often placed on the yoni. It is this musky odor that must
be called to mind. The yoni has its own fresh, soft flavor, the
essence of the female. This soft musk taste is a most powerful
mind stimulant.

The sound of the yoni is next experienced. Many find this
difficult to achieve at first. It is the sound of the heartbeat, the
hollow deep drum rhythm that can occasionally be heard when
a large bass drum is very gently tapped. It is a slow rhythm, an
earth rhythm, that pulses with life.

Lastly the whole feeling of the yoni is experienced: the
mother, the lover, and the nymph feeling combined into one. It
is both pleasure and pain. Through mutual understanding, both
partners perfect their yonic caresses. This meditation can bring
each partner to the point of orgasm. At this point a single touch
of the (artificial) phallus should push the yogin into orgasm. The
intent of the meditation is to get to the point of orgasm and stay
there.

Shakti and Shiva

If you stem-meditate on your partner, he or she will come to
you; then both will ascend. Each needs the other to gain release.
Until you welcome that represented by your partner and under-

stand it, nothing will work. Those who regularly practice this stem meditation open up their consciousness to the forces of their partner. You gain more understanding of each other and what he/she represents. You can carry this meditation on to include other aspects of the characteristics your partner represents. Thus your consciousness is expanded. See the God-ess principles within you, and they will grow stronger.

Maithuna Training for Men

During the Tantric ritual of Maithuna, Male A's lingam is within Male B's posterior yoni, but ejaculation is forbidden. Male B lies on his back; his legs are intertwined with Male A's. Male A enters Male B very deeply and solidly while lying on his side. Proceed with the rest of the instructions on page 78.

Maithuna Training for Women

During the Tantric ritual of Maithuna, Female A has the phallus inserted into Female B's yoni as well as her own. Female B lies on her back; her legs are intertwined with Female A's. Female A enters Female B very deeply and solidly while lying on her side. Proceed with the rest of the instructions on page 78.

NOTES FOR CHAPTER 5

When two men do the basic exercise on page 108, a male is in the lower position; so when gay males do this, each man should have a turn on the bottom. Male A sits somewhat forward on Male B, who is on his back. Male B rotates his pelvis so that the lingam alternately reaches a high inside the posterior yoni and is almost completely extracted from the posterior yoni. As each male learns to rotate the pelvis more, his partner must lift himself up from him because Male A will be able to remove the lingam completely from the posterior yoni in the downward rotation, interrupting the exercise.

The basic exercise is easy to adapt for lesbian Tantrists. Each woman can take a turn as the top and as the bottom, thereby gaining the pleasures and benefits of both positions. No artificial phallus is necessary here. Follow the rest of the instructions on page 108 onward, but delete lingam references.

Rising Sun and Moon

For both men and women, the directions for the rising sun and moon exercise on page 108 are followed just as described in the book. Instead of male/female, read male/male or female/female. Again, maximum enjoyment comes from switching positions. This also applies to the Eclipse (page 109), the Rocking Chair (page 110), and Riding (page 111).

The Cobra and the Swan

Because the insertion of the lingam into the yoni is not required for this exercise (page 110), no adaptation is required. If the women desire, the artificial phallus is used. This would be more difficult for males due to the lifting. It is suggested you do this exercise without insertion first to get the hang of it.

Circle of Completeness for Men

When the circle coupling is arranged, each Male A lies on his side and each Male B lies on his back. Male A's lingam crosses Male B's lingam at a sideways angle. The next couple connects in the same way so that Male A may caress the face of the next Male B and kiss his head and chest. From here, follow the remainder of the instructions.

Circle of Completeness for Women

Female A lies on her side and inserts one end of the phallus into her yoni; then the other end of the phallus is inserted into Female B's yoni at a sideways angle.

NOTES FOR CHAPTER 6

Chivalry and Gallantry

Just as with heterosexuals, courtesy and kindness are important and proper with gay men and women. You should always be ready to protect your partner when on an outing. Likewise there is nothing wrong with opening and holding the door for your partner. It is also good to enter into new areas together, supporting each other. Treat each other with the affection you enjoy.

The Maithuna Ritual

In the period after the meal of the great monthly welcoming festival (page 125), Partner B worships Partner A. Partner B caresses Partner A and does any grooming that needs doing. Partner A is oiled and massaged and made as god-like as can be. The same applies to gay men and women partners. Then proceed with the festival as explained in the chapter.

Ritual Copulation for Men

During the eight days following the moon festival (Maithuna Ritual), each partner carefully arouses the other until both are close to orgasm. The lingam of Male A is inserted into the posterior yoni of Male B in any desired sex position. Both partners come quickly to orgasm and remain coupled thereafter until the tension is released. This ritual occurs in Male A's sleeping area and each partner then returns to his respective bed to sleep. It is an honor to be invited to a partner's room.

Ritual Copulation for Women

During the eight days following the moon festival (the Maithuna Ritual), each partner carefully arouses the other until both are close to orgasm. Female A inserts the artificial phallus; then the lingam is inserted into Female B's yoni in any desired sex position. Both partners come quickly to orgasm and remain coupled thereafter until the tensions are released. This ritual copulation occurs in Female A's sleeping area and each partner returns to her own bed to sleep.

The Kundalini Circle

The Great Full Moon Festival is the reverse of the Great Monthly Welcoming Festival. Partner A is totally subservient to Partner B. Any grooming Partner B wants, he or she gets, and the same with services. Partner B is worshipped, massaged, oiled, and petted.

Note that whoever is Partner A at the beginning of the moon cycle remains so for the whole cycle. When a new yearly cycle begins or when assigned a new partner, roles may be changed.

NOTES FOR CHAPTER 8

Maithunic Marriage

Following instructions on page 163, the group comes together in a huddle in the center of the exercise room. Now they enter into the most sacred part of the rite, as the couples are going to become married for a month.

Men: After the kiss is exchanged, they lie on the floor with Male A on Male B's right side. Male A lies on his left side and Male B turns his head so he can look into his eyes while lying on his back. Gently Male A lifts Male B's left leg over his legs and brings his lingam against the posterior yoni by scissoring Male B's right leg between his own legs. Male B's left leg rests on Male A's right hip. Male B reaches down and inserts the lingam into the posterior yoni. They quietly lie in this position for 32 minutes. Follow the remainder of the instructions in the chapter.

Women: After the kiss is exchanged, they lie on the floor with Female A on Female B's right side. Female A lies on her left side and Female B turns her head so she can look into her eyes while she lies on her back. Gently Female A lifts Female B's left leg over her legs and (after inserting one end of the phallus into her yoni) brings the other end of the phallus against Female B's yoni by scissoring Female B's right leg between her own legs. Female B's left leg rests on Female A's right hip. Female B reaches down and inserts the phallus into her yoni. They lie quietly in this position for 32 minutes. Follow the remainder of the instructions in the chapter.

Ritual for Activating the Pelvic Chakra for Men

Before the ritual, be sure sufficient lubricant has been applied to the posterior yoni. As instructed on page 168, everyone stands in a tight circle after preparation and proceeds with the chant and motions.

The motion is kept up for several minutes until it is obvious that all members are ready and eager for sexual contact. The leading Male B breaks the circle and grabs the lingam of the Male A to his right, and pumps it quite violently. The other Male B's immediately follow his example. The Male A's fall to the floor with the Male B's on top of them. Each Male B tears off Male A's loincloth and forces the posterior yoni down over the lingam in a fairly violent motion. Each Male B holds his body vertical. He does not lower himself onto Male A in a loving manner. He moves violently upward and downward for eight strokes, then breaks off the encounter. Each Male B moves clockwise to the next Male A and treats him in the same way. At this stage no one reaches climax, though the Male B's remain ravening and violent.

In the second round of contacts, each Male B becomes more cunning in his actions. He is more coy and more gentle. Now when Male B approaches Male A, Male A throws him on his back and thrusts into him. Male B scratches and bites. Male A responds by kissing him violently while continuing the thrusts until he climaxes. But Male B is not yet satisfied. He wants it again. With all his wiles he works on Male A's lingam until it is hard again and he is inside him once more.

One of Rakini's weapons is a whip. Many houses allow its use to encourage and rouse Male A. Male B must have him again before the ritual ends. Male B can be as loving now as he wants, but he will not be denied.

The point of understanding of the chakra occurs at the instant before reaching climax. At this instant Male A may try to withdraw, but Male B forces continuation. It is in this attempted withdrawal and forced continuation that the chakra is finally entered.

Ritual for Activating the Pelvic Chakra for Women

As instructed on page 168, everyone stands in a tight circle after preparation and proceeds with the chant and motions. The motion is kept up for several minutes until it is obvious that all members are ready and eager for sexual contact. The leading Female B breaks the circle and grabs the phallus already inserted in Female A's (to her right) yoni, and pumps it quite violently. The other Female B's immediately follow her example. The Female A's fall to the floor with the Female B's on top of them. Each Female B tears off Female A's loincloth and forces the yoni over the phallus in a violent motion, so violent that in some houses lubricant is applied to the yoni of all partners before the ritual. Each Female B holds her body vertical. She does not lower herself onto Female A in a loving manner. She moves violently upward and downward for eight strokes, then breaks off the encounter. Each Female B moves clockwise to the next Female A and treats her in the same way. At this stage no one reaches climax, though the Female B's remain ravening and violent.

In the second round of contacts, each Female B becomes more cunning in her actions. She is more coy and more gentle.

Now when Female B approaches Female A, Female A throws her on her back and thrusts with the phallus into her. Female B scratches and bites. Female A responds by kissing her violently while continuing the thrusts until she climaxes. But Female B is not yet satisfied. She wants it again. With all her wiles she works on Female A's yoni with the still inserted phallus until she senses Female A's arousal. Then Female B inserts the other end of the phallus inside her once more.

One of Rakini's weapons is a whip. Many houses allow its use to encourage and rouse Female A. Female B must have her again before the ritual ends. Female B can be as loving now as she wants, but she will not be denied.

The point of understanding of the chakra occurs at the instant before reaching climax. At this instant Female A may try to withdraw, but Female B forces continuation. It is in this attempted withdrawal and forced continuation that the chakra is finally entered.

Pelvic Chakra Activation— Guided Meditation

This meditation occurs after the ritual. It is a stem lingam/yoni meditation. The first phase is to do a deep and complete meditation on your partner's sexual equipment. In other words, males meditate on the lingam and females meditate on the yoni. The male emphasis is on the erect lingam starting with the state of erection that results from long unfulfilled need for sexual satisfaction. The female emphasis is on the erect nipples and clitoris also resulting from long unfulfilled need for sexual satisfaction.

Navel Chakra

To activate the navel chakra read "yogi" as Male A or Female A, and "yogin" as Male B or Female B. Then proceed with instructions on page 176. The yogi chant should be as deep as possible without straining, and likewise the yogin chant as high a pitch as possible without straining. The posterior yoni remains the male yoni, and the phallus remains the female lingam.

Throat Chakra

In the ritual for activating the throat chakra (page 190), substitute Male A or Female A for "yogi" and Male B or Female B for "yogin."

Brow Chakra

Element: The element of the chakra is life force. This is a superior form of water. A new thought creation has been formed from your union. Although with gay Tantrists pregnancy cannot occur, you can be aware of a special feeling between you—your two life forces as one.

Animal: The traditional animal image of the chakra is the coupled partners. They are coupled standing up so their bodies form a vertical, symbolic yin-yang. The image of the tiny seedling of a flowering tree remains the more modern image, as mentioned in the chapter.

Goddess: The skull in Shakti's hand reminds you once more of your mortality and that you must create new life before leaving this plane of existence. New human life does not occur with the gay Tantrist, so a substitute should be utilized. The planting, nurturing, and caring from seed of a fruit tree are one way you may satisfy this. You alone will be responsible for one special tree and see that it brings forth its fruit so all can enjoy. After you have helped in creating new life, Shakti will grant you the boon of understanding spiritual life.

Ritual for Activating the Brow Chakra

Men: Follow the instructions given (page 197), but make the following adaptations: When the last garment is removed, the OM is very loud. Male A mounts Male B and pulls Male A's lingam into his posterior yoni, reaching down for the buttocks and firmly pulling Male A down onto him while lotusing upward to receive him. Full copulation occurs. It must be a firm and satisfying experience for both partners.

While fertilization cannot occur, nevertheless at the instant of mutual orgasm, the image of new life in its lustrous whiteness, its warmth and pinkness, must be held by both partners. After this, proceed with the mind-melding discussed on page 198.

Women: When the last garment is removed, the O<u>M</u> is very loud. Female A, with phallus inserted, mounts Female B. Female B pulls the lingam into herself, reaching down for the buttocks and firmly pulling Female A down onto herself while she lotuses upward to receive her. Full copulation occurs. It must be a firm and satisfying experience for both participants.

Everyone realizes that fertilization cannot occur, but at the instant of mutual orgasm, the image of new life in its lustrous whiteness, its warmth and pinkness, must be held by both partners. After this, proceed with the mind-melding described on page 198.

NOTES FOR CHAPTER 9

Throat Chakra

Follow the directions in the chapter (page 222), except that the mantra HO<u>M</u> is started in a higher pitched singing by all partners. Then as the pitch is lowered and after eight repetitions, the final chant is done in a voice as deep and low as possible.

Pelvic Chakra

Read "yogi" as Male A or Female A and "yogin" as Male B or Female B. After more cuddling and kissing, the ritual should be handled as follows for men: Male B introduces Male A's lingam into his posterior yoni while Male A remains on his side. As before, they touch each other except in the areas of the lingam or the posterior yoni. From here complete the ritual as written in the chapter (page 240).

Women will complete this ritual as follows: Female B introduces Female A's phallus into her yoni while Female A remains on her side. As before, they touch each other except in the area of the yoni, though they can make sexual movements with contractions of the yoni. From here complete the ritual as written in the chapter.

NOTES FOR APPENDIX 1

The Mare and the Hare

With women, the size of the yoni is not an inhibiting factor because artificial phalli come in various sizes and a double-ended one can be easily adapted for gay female partners. However, with men, the hare, bull, and horse divisions should still be given a certain amount of consideration. The most equal divisions are hare/hare, hare/bull, bull/bull, bull/horse, and horse/horse. This would be a matter for each house to discuss and set up regulations for admitting new members, but this is something that is up to those involved to set limits or not.

The Dyadic Couple

Selfishness has no place in the Tantrist house. If you have reached orgasm and your partner has not, selflessness means staying with your partner until he or she has also reached orgasm, or assist when your partner is ready. Each must give physical support and help to the other.

BIBLIOGRAPHY

Avalon, A., tr. *Tantra of the Great Liberation*. New York: Dover, 1972.

Bharati, A. *Tantric Tradition*. Garden City, NY: Anchor/ Doubleday, 1970.

Billion, A. *Kundalini: Secrets of Ancient Yoga*. New York: Prentice-Hall, 1982.

Blofeld, J. *Tantric Mysticism of Tibet*. New York: Causeway Books, 1968.

Burton, R., tr. *The Kama Sutra*. New York: Medical Press, 1962.

Chang, J. *Tao of Love and Sex*. New York: E.P. Dutton, 1977.

Eliade, Mircea. *Yoga: Immortality and Freedom*. Princeton, NJ: Princeton University Press, 1970.

Garrison, O. *Tantra: The Yoga of Sex*. New York: Julian Press/ Crown, 1983.

Johnston, C. *Yoga Sutras of Patanjali*. Albuquerque, NM: Brotherhood of Life, 1983.

Lewis, J. *Yoga for Couples*. Brookline, MA: Autumn Press, 1979.

Michell, J. *New View over Atlantis*. New York: E.P. Dutton, 1984.

Mumford, Dr. J. *Ectasy through Tantra*. St. Paul, MN: Llewellyn, 1988.

Pagal Baba. *Temple of the Phallic King*. New York: Simon & Schuster, 1973.

Prabhavananda, Swami, and C. Isherwood, trs. *The Bhagavad-Gita: The Song of God*. Hollywood, CA: Vedanta Press, 1987.

Radha, S. *Kundalini Yoga for the West*. Boston: Shambhala, 1981.

Rawson, P. *Art of Tantra*. New York: Thames & Hudson, 1985.

Richmond, S. *How to Be Healthy with Yoga*. New York: Arc Books, 1962.

Sen, K.M. *Hinduism*. New York: Penquin, 1984.

Singh, M. *Himalayan Art.* New York: Macmillan, 1971.

Stone, M. *When God Was a Woman.* San Diego, CA: Dial Press, 1976.

Tucci, G. *Theory and Practice of the Mandala.* York Beach, ME: Samuel Weiser, 1970. Now out of print.

Wood, E. *Yoga.* New York: Penquin, 1968.

QUESTIONNAIRE

This questionnaire is designed for those who

- are interested in furthering the great work of Tantra Yoga;
- have completed some of the exercises in the book;
- are interested in founding or joining a house.

To discourage thrill-seekers, we need you to answer the following questions before we put your name on our network list.

Name_____

Social Security Number_____

Address_____

_____

_____

Marital Status _____ (single, married, living together, widowed, other)

Sexual Preference _____ (same gender, opposite gender, both)

Age_____ Gender_____ Height_____ Weight_____
General Health_____

You consider yourself to be a   hare   / /   deer   / /

                                   bull   / /   mare   / /

                                   horse / /   elephant / /

Financial Status: Annual Income $_____ Assets _____
Liabilities _____

On separate sheets of paper:

1. In your own words describe the highest chakra you have reached.

2. Complete Table 1 which has been reproduced for you on the back of this form.

3. Suggest a technique through which eight adults (four male, four female) or their gay equivalents can completely meld with one another.

4. Should people of different colored skins have separate houses, or should they be part of an integrated house? Explain your answer.

5. Write a creation myth "from above" and "from below."

Table 1. Maximizing Your Force

Hour of Day	Weak			Average			Strong		
	1	2	3	1	2	3	1	2	3
1 A.M.									
3 A.M.									
5 A.M.									
7 A.M.									
9 A.M.									
11 A.M.									
1 P.M.									
3 P.M.									
5 P.M.									
7 P.M.									
9 P.M.									
11 P.M.